THE CONTENTED VEGAN

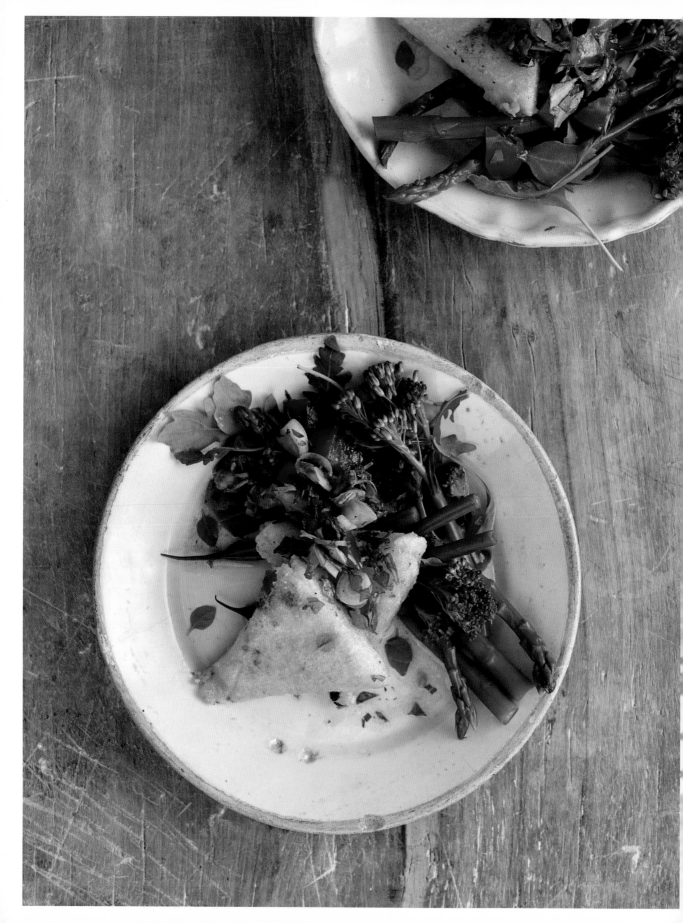

THE
CONTENTED
VEGAN

Recipes and philosophy
from a family kitchen

PEGGY BRUSSEAU

To the power of green and the abundance of nature;
with love and gratitude to my three menfolk.

First published in 2021 by Head of Zeus Ltd.

975312468

A CIP catalogue record for this book is available from the British Library.

ISBN (HB): 9781838934682
ISBN (E): 9781838934705

Printed in China

Head of Zeus Ltd
5–8 Hardwick Street
London EC1R 4RG
headofzeus.com

Designed and produced for
Head of Zeus by Unipress Books Ltd

Stay in touch with Peggy and lots of vegan resources at her website, PeggyBrusseau.com

RECIPE NOTES

Unless stated otherwise, each recipe is designed to serve 4 people a moderate portion size. There are no 'super-size' dishes included, though there are many that provide enough for second helpings!

Most ingredients are very easy to find, but a few will need you to try a grocer who sells ingredients for cuisines from other world regions. I have called these 'ethnic' or 'neighbourhood' grocers. I use these grocers in my area because they sell unusual and fascinating food items that serve the needs of various religions, immigrant/ethnic communities and world cuisines. The proprietors give helpful advice if I don't know how an item is used and will get stock in for me if I ask – I always learn something new!

All preparation times are approximate.

Fresh produce should be thoroughly washed before use.

Bracketed terms are intended for American readers.

Where spoon and cup measures are given, these are standard spoon measures and standard US cups:

1 teaspoon = 5ml
1 tablespoon = 15ml*
1 US cup = 240ml

*Australian standard tablespoons are 20ml, therefore Australian readers should use 3 teaspoons in place of a tablespoon for measuring small quantities.

Spoon and cup measures are level unless stated otherwise.

Ovens can vary: always refer to the manufacturer's instructions.

CONTENTS

INTRODUCTION

WELCOME

For the past thirty years I have eaten and prepared only vegan food. During that time I enjoyed two healthy pregnancies followed by periods of breastfeeding and – with my husband – raised two strong, athletic sons who continue to be vegan. Throughout those years I daily provided bountiful plant-based meals, at very little cost, for family and any friends who happened to drop by. But in the beginning, it wasn't easy.

Back in those far-off days, 'vegan' wasn't a word we used much. To be vegetarian was unusual enough, but to be vegan … It sounded pretty eccentric. There wasn't much information available – and what was available wasn't always helpful. Recipes were worthy but often dull. Restaurants and even friends needed prior notification of our food preferences before we came for dinner. We were cross-examined by friends, family and sometimes health professionals on the wisdom of our diet: Did we know what we were doing?

In fact, yes. We had to know what we were doing. Not just for our own sakes, but for our growing children. We went out of our way to learn everything we needed to know about vegan nutrition; about the ethical and philosophical arguments in favour of veganism; and, of course, about ways of making vegan food that had meat-eaters salivating.

While at first it felt as if we were swimming against the current, now it seems the tide has turned. A plant-based way of eating is gaining in popularity, and for very good reasons. Eating a vegan diet is not hard work. It does not even feel like giving something up. It feels like letting go of something that has burdened you, so that you can hold on to something that is truly precious. Choosing a plant-based way of eating, even for a short time, gives you a jolt of pure life force. Health, mood and outlook improve. Levels of mental and physical energy increase. And while shifting to a vegan diet is good for you personally, it is even better for our planet.

Eating lower in the food chain takes the pressure off our world's natural resources. It has a hugely positive effect on some of the most important environmental issues of our time, including tropical deforestation, the survival of indigenous peoples and even climate change. In short, if you care about the future of life on Earth, going vegan is one of the smartest choices you can make.

What a pleasant way to make a difference! Because preparing vegan meals is a delight. Daily contact with food plants is grounding and healing, and the sense of connection with natural abundance is uplifting. A relaxed exploration of the diverse textures, flavours and aromas of the meals you make is a journey into creativity. I would love to share my experiences, knowledge and recipes with you in the coming pages.

Peggy xx

MAKING THE SWITCH

As far back as the so-called hunter-gatherer phase of human existence, plants have provided the day-to-day subsistence that has enabled humankind to come this far. Although the practice of eating a plant-based diet has existed for centuries, the word that currently defines it – vegan – was devised in Britain in 1944. Its creation has been attributed to Donald Watson, a founder member of the Vegan Society. He said the word 'vegan' was created 'from the first and last letters of "VEGetariAN" because the diet grew out of vegetarianism and was seen as its natural conclusion'.

While we know a growing number of people are choosing to eat a vegan diet, the reasons why they choose it vary. Generally, though, these fall into four broad categories.

* Environment – they realize that eating a plant-based diet will help to reduce the severity of environmental problems
* Vegetarianism – they see switching to veganism as a natural progression from their current vegetarian diet
* Health – they either want to preserve their good health or have health problems they have heard the vegan diet might help to resolve
* Ethics and animal welfare – they see that exploitation of animals is inhumane and they no longer wish to support its practice by eating animal-based foods

Whichever reason first inspires a switch to a plant-based way of eating, after a while people start making connections they hadn't made before. New realizations come to the surface that have their own momentum within each individual. Perhaps this is because veganism is not only a practical decision, but a choice that touches on the inner life of a person as well. People who have transitioned to a plant-based diet report feeling better about themselves as often as they report feeling healthier in themselves.

There is a simplicity about the vegan way of eating that seems to help cast off not just excess pounds and health problems, but habits and patterns that burden the thinking and feeling life, too. This makes sense when you see that the vegan diet is based on food choices that show consideration for other life forms. The vegan diet excludes any foods or products made from the body of an animal. This means the fat, flesh or skin of any animal, fish or bird, as well as their bones, blood, eggs or milk. Many vegans also do not eat honey (see page 36). Acting from the heart as well as the intellect can have beneficial, even profound consequences for the whole person.

Often people seek support for their choice and answers to their deeper questions by exploring what others have said or written in connection with food choices. The topic arises with surprising frequency in general conversation and in areas of study such as ethics, social history and religion. Pulled together, these discussions represent a philosophical platform for the vegan way of life. They support veganism not as a passing fad, but as a well-considered way of life that has endured over many centuries and now is being widely adopted.

THE 80/20 RULE

Switching to a plant-based diet needn't be daunting; you can begin to amend your food choices right now, but you don't have to do it all at once! Making the switch should be low-stress, delicious and feel personal to you. Be patient and take your time. There is no better way to start than by using this gentle rule.

The 80/20 rule is very simple: approximately 80 per cent of your diet is already likely to be plant-based and only the remaining 20 per cent needs adjusting. Check it out for yourself – recall what you ate last week and see how it measures up. For example:

* That burger you ate last Tuesday might have been beef, but the chips, the bun and most of the fillings were largely, if not entirely, plant-based.
* You might pour cow's milk over your muesli every morning, but the muesli, its topping of berries and the orange juice you sip with it are all plant-based.

A few simple adjustments to the ingredients of almost any meal can make it vegan. Change that beef burger to a bean burger, use plant milk on your muesli, and you instantly turn two daily meals into vegan meals with almost no effort. If you can firmly establish 80 per cent of your diet as plant-based and work on adjusting the remaining 20 per cent, very soon your diet will be totally vegan.

The 80/20 rule can be used for the long term, too. For instance, although much of what you eat will be vegan, not all of it will be as freshly prepared, carefully sourced and rich in whole foods as you'd like. Perhaps meals out and social gatherings feel problematic. Well, they needn't be. Rather than refuse the invitation, lean back on the rule. Accept the invitation, have a vegan meal out including imported or refined foods, and feel good about yourself. If all or most of your diet is plant-based and you aim for 80 per cent of that to meet your ideals, you are doing brilliantly.

There will always be scope for improvements or adjustments. I enjoy this – it means that I can explore and discover, for instance, what changes I can make to 20 per cent of my spice purchases or to 20 per cent of the household products I buy. The 80/20 rule can help you to discover which of the plant-based foods already in your diet can be 'upgraded' for any reason, but especially to increase the variety of plants you consume. Variety in your diet is crucial to good nutrition and naturally builds 'local' (see page 12) and 'in season' (see page 14) into your way of eating, too.

Having introduced the 80/20 rule, it's vital to remember that eating a vegan diet is an individual's choice. There are no vegan enforcement officers in the back room waiting to drag you into the street if you put a forbidden food to your lips. The decision is all yours. The benefits extend beyond you.

LET FOOD BE YOUR MEDICINE

It's important to understand that deciding to become vegan does not automatically guarantee a healthy diet – but it's very simple to create one. Building a nutrient-rich diet that supports optimal health for you, your family and the environment centres on four key ideas:

* Eat plant-based foods that are as whole (unprocessed) as possible
* Choose organically and/or locally grown produce where possible
* Select produce that is in season, if possible
* Eat a wide variety of foods each day

In the 5th century BCE, the physician Hippocrates (often seen as the father of medicine) observed that daily 'doses' of nutrient-rich fresh food had a cumulative, beneficial effect on health; and that daily doses of poor-quality food had a cumulative – but opposite – effect. Hippocrates taught his pupils that a simple diet, comprised of the many locally grown vegetables, fruits, nuts, oils, herbs and whole grains, would preserve health by preventing illness. If a person did become ill, that way of eating would also restore good health swiftly. The guidance 'Let food be your medicine and your medicine be your food' is attributed to him.

Roll the clock forward twenty-five centuries and it is pretty clear that he got it right. After decades of understating the relevance of diet to health, modern medical science is gradually acknowledging its powerful influence. Cancer, the degenerative and auto-immune diseases, heart disease, diabetes and obesity are all responsive to changes in diet. So are allergies, migraines, insomnia, hyperactivity and premenstrual syndrome, to name a few. You already know for yourself that what you eat makes a difference to how you feel. So it seems sensible to devise a delicious diet that will steer you, day after day, toward optimal health.

A varied diet of whole, plant-based foods provides essential nutrients in beneficial doses that are naturally present in the food. It is now known that these nutrients come with powerful companions: a variety of bioactive compounds called 'phytochemicals' (*phyto* means 'plant'). These act synergistically with the essential vitamins and minerals already present, to reduce the potential for an excess effect of any one nutrient. Synergy, where the whole is greater than the sum of its parts, is the perfect term to describe this phenomenon. It means that the plant has it all figured out; its components naturally influence each other to create nutritional poise.

Using the 80/20 rule, gradually turn 80 per cent of your diet into your phytochemical 'medicine chest' by following the four key ideas outlined above. Let the remaining 20 per cent include:

* Fortified foods that augment nutrient groups, such as yeast products rich in B_{12}
* Non-locally grown, ethnic and global foods that allow exploration and social ease, such as olive oil, avocado, tropical fruit and exotic spices, grains and legumes.

THE MEANING OF 'WHOLE'

A 'whole' food remains largely unprocessed, with all or most of its plant material retained and its complement of nutrients available to you: it's an 'unbroken' food. Processed or refined foods are 'broken'. Parts of the plant with significant nutritional value are removed, usually because their presence makes it hard to store the food for long periods – an example of commercial interests being at odds with consumer health.

Refinement can degrade nutrient value to the point of creating 'empty' foods, which have a calorie count but little or no nutritional value. For example, a refined grain is usually white. The whiteness is the starchy endosperm of the grain, meant to provide all the fuel the grain (or seed) needs to grow into a plant. The fact that it is exposed means that the outer layers of bran have been removed and discarded. What a pity! These layers are rich in fibre, B vitamins and numerous phytochemicals, such as antioxidants. But that's not all; the germ, which was discarded with the bran, exists right at the heart of a grain. As the potential plant, it is a powerhouse of nutrients. That tiny germ carries the life force – but it, too, has been removed. Up to 90 per cent of the grain's nutritional value will have been lost in the refinement process.

A diet based on refined foods will give you enough calories each day, but it is much more difficult to obtain adequate nourishment. Although you have eaten, your body continues to seek nutrients because they are the substances that make you feel well and that keep you healthy. So, you keep eating. If you continue to eat highly processed food, weight gain, even obesity, could easily result – and you would still be undernourished.

FORTIFICATION AND SUPPLEMENTS

Food producers do make an effort to 'add back' nutrients that will increase the nutritional value of their refined product. This is one form (but not the best!) of fortification. To make it work requires additional ingredients such as preservatives, colourants, flavour enhancers, fillers and binders. The result is a product that is uniform, easy to package and will have a long shelf life. But it's still broken.

The parts of the food that were refined away will be sold on – often to you as, for instance, bran to sprinkle on your cereal. But, in such a case, one half plus one half does not make one whole. You cannot put the parts back together again. In the course of refinement, vital nutrients are lost that cannot be replaced, not even by fortification. Meanwhile, taking supplements of nutrients, isolated after extraction from their source food plant, is observed to have a weak or inconsistent protective effect compared to when they are consumed as part of a 'whole' food. In addition, the long-term safety and efficacy of isolated nutrient supplements require more study.

The way out of a refined food spiral is to select one or two foods that you already enjoy and decide you will eat them in their whole form. For instance, try wholegrain brown rice or unpeeled potatoes, cooked however you like. Then, use the 80/20 rule to move toward a whole-food pattern of eating … gradually and with ease.

THE IMPORTANCE OF LOCAL

Imagine you are a neolithic forager, picking from the woodlands and verges as you walk. Well hidden over there is a sweet root and next to it a leafy plant with a tangy flavour. Further along are young apples and, as you stretch to get a few, you notice that the brambles catching at your tunic will soon be heavy with blackberries. When you arrive back at your settlement, you carry the root, a pouch full of leaves and an apple or two. The rest is gone and your belly is full. You've been nibbling and sampling – discovering the bounty that is all around you.

Truly fresh food is newly harvested – your neolithic ancestor couldn't have had a fresher meal. In modern times, everything about that meal would be marketed as 'ultra' or 'super' or 'mega' because the flavours and colours would be strong and distinct, while the textures would be those of a vital, healthy plant.

Crucially, the nutrient value of each food item would be far greater than the value of a similar meal foraged today. Notable studies have shown a significant decline in nutrient values of fruits and vegetables over the past fifty years. This loss is largely attributed to changes in farming practices that have led to greatly reduced soil quality. The plants cannot assimilate nutrients that aren't there in the soil – and, if those nutrients aren't in the plants, we can't get them either.

Alongside this issue, the modern practice of harvesting foods before they are ripe diminishes the nutrients that reach your plate. These not-quite-ready-to-eat foods are often shipped huge distances to sell to consumers in other regions. This further reduces nutrient value and increases the cost of the food, sometimes by up to 80 per cent. To ensure the underripe, long-distance food reaches the shelves in edible form, foods are often 'treated' using costly products or procedures.

Flavour, colour, texture and nutrient value are markers of a food's quality. These qualities are determined by the health of the plant and the soil in which it grows. The moment a plant is harvested it is removed from its source of nutrients and begins to lose quality. You and I notice this and say, 'That isn't fresh.'

Modern food production includes methods for simulating freshness that do nothing to prevent nutrient loss. These practices include: immersion in chlorine baths to inhibit surface bacteria; application of waxes to inhibit loss of moisture; inhibition of the ripening process by adjustments in temperature; and use of ethylene gas to promote ripening. Such practices are used for the extended storage and shipping of fruits and vegetables – especially those from other climate regions.

The most obvious reason for loss of quality is time. Your neolithic forager enjoyed maximum nutrient value and quality because almost no time passed between harvesting and eating.

To maximize the quality of the fruit and vegetables you eat, bring one or more of these simple steps into your way of shopping:

* Buy from farmers' markets in your vicinity. It is very enjoyable to find and get to know local growers and to learn what's 'coming up' in the harvesting calendar.
* Find markets or grocers that draw their produce from within a radius of 100 kilometres (60 miles). That distance can be travelled easily within one day, which means your produce is likely to have been harvested that morning or the previous afternoon. If in doubt, ask!
* Find an organic or biodynamic grower and buy what they produce. Their growing and gardening practices usually include naturally enriched soils that deliver more nutrients.
* Subscribe to a 'box delivery' service. These provide a box of in-season, locally grown (and often organic) fruit and vegetables on a weekly or biweekly basis, delivered to your door.
* Find local or neighbourhood gardeners who are willing to sell or share their homegrown produce.
* Plant your own garden! Use your patio, balcony or windowsill, and grow what you can.

Local is best for other reasons as well:

* You will be supporting the local economy, creating a sense of community and building a network of people who also care about your locale.
* You will be reducing the need for preservatives and packaging.
* You will be helping to reduce the cost and environmental impact of food transport.

There is no single agreed definition of 'local', but there is a definite *feeling* of what comprises your neighbourhood, your part of the world. This is true of both plants and people. Food plants that are grown locally to where you live (especially if grown organically) are likely to be a good match for you. As you share the same climate and the same seasons, the nutrients they provide will come at a time of year when they will be of most benefit to you.

THE BEAUTY OF SEASONS

You know how it goes. Spring loiters beneath patches of grubby snow and under mouldering piles of leaves, waiting for the Earth to tilt around the corner of its orbit. Then, rather suddenly, the new season arrives: green and balmy. We are ready for it, can hardly wait for sunny weekends, salads and lighter clothing. The months roll on into summer warmth and long, sunlit evenings: the parks are full, the pavements (sidewalks) are crowded. Everyone is out collecting sunlight and storing it in their cells.

At the end of summer, the Earth opens its arms and displays its generosity. Food plants are ripening and plumping, and all in such abundance. This is a glut – extra to requirements. If you have a garden, you may feel that you can't keep up. But there is another mood, a whisper, reminding you to save some for later. The adage 'Waste not, want not' comes from this time of year: until very recently, people had to prepare for winter by purposefully storing their food at the end of summer and early in the autumn (fall). If they didn't do that, they went hungry.

These days, the harvesting and storage are done on a massive scale and in an industrialized manner. We can just go to the supermarket and buy whatever we want or need, at any time of year, which can create a sense that the seasons do not matter. They do matter. It's just that the link between food and seasons has become obscured, for urban dwellers especially. When you eat foods in the season in which they ripen, you are more likely to:

* eat locally grown food, with all the environmental, social and health benefits that brings
* enjoy foods with greater nutrient value and more freshness, flavour, colour and texture
* naturally and easily increase the variety of foods in your diet, one of the fundamentals
* derive more benefit from phytochemicals in the food
* find that foods are cheaper than if purchased out of season

In your kitchen, the change of season can inspire the planting of fresh herbs on your windowsill, arranging a picnic, or preparing warm, aromatic meals to make everyone feel at home. Acknowledging the seasons gives us reasons to try new dishes and new styles of cooking. It is the original solution to the boredom of too-often-repeated meals, as there is always something new coming up.

Of course, it can be a real treat to sample exotic fruits and unusual ingredients out of season and from far-flung parts of the world. Enjoy those foods, and appreciate all that is involved in bringing them to your plate. For the rest of the time, it is as much fun to explore food that is in season where you live. To get started, make use of seasonal food lists, talk to local gardeners and use the 80/20 rule to gradually bring a little more fresh and nutritious seasonal produce into your diet.

SEASONAL PRODUCE

SPRING	SUMMER		AUTUMN		WINTER
Asparagus	Apricots	Lemon balm	Apples	Leeks	Apples
Broccoli	Asparagus	Lettuce	Aubergines	Lemon balm	Bay leaves
Carrots	Aubergines	Loganberries	(eggplants)	Lettuce	Beetroot (beets)
Cauliflower	(eggplants)	Lovage	Basil	Loganberries	Brussels sprouts
Celeriac	Basil	Mangetout	Beetroot (beets)	Lovage	Cabbage
(celery root)	Beetroot (beets)	(snow peas)	Bilberries	Marjoram	Carrot
Celery	Blueberries	Marjoram	Blackberries	Marrow (summer	Cauliflower
Chicory	Borage	Melon	Blackcurrants	squash)	Celeriac
Cucumbers	Borlotti	Mint	Blueberries	Medlar	(celery root)
Curly kale	(cranberry)	Mulberries	Borage	Mint	Celery
Elderflowers	beans	Nasturtium	Brussels sprouts	Mulberries	Chicory
Gooseberries	Broad beans	Nettles	Cabbage	Nasturtium	Cranberries
Mint	(fava beans)	New potatoes	Carrots	Nettles	Fennel
Nettle	Broccoli	Onions	Cauliflower	Onions	(finocchio)
New potatoes	Cabbage	Oregano	Cavolo nero	Oranges	Jerusalem
Onions	Carrots	Pak choi	Celeriac	Oregano	artichokes
Oranges	Cauliflower	(bok choy)	(celery root)	Parsley	Kale
Parsley	Chard	Parsley	Celery	Parsnips	Kohlrabi
Purple sprouting	(silver beet)	Peaches	Chard	Pears	Leeks
broccoli	Cherries	Peppers	(silver beet)	Plums	Medlars
Radishes	Chervil	(capsicums)	Chervil	Potatoes	Onions
Rhubarb	Chillies	Plums	Chestnuts	Pumpkins	Oranges
Savoy cabbage	Chives	Potatoes	Chicory	Quinces	Parsley
Shallots	Coriander	Radishes	Chillies	Rocket (arugula)	Parsnips
Sorrel	(cilantro)	Raspberries	Chives	Romanesco	Passion fruit
Spinach	Courgettes	Rhubarb	Coriander	broccoli	Pears
Spring greens	(zucchini)	Rocket (arugula)	(cilantro)	Rosemary	Potatoes
(collard greens)	Courgette	Rosemary	Courgettes	Sage	Quinces
Spring onions	(zucchini) flowers	Runner beans	(zucchini)	Salsify (oyster	Red cabbage
(scallions)	Cucumber	Sage	Cranberries	plant)	Romanesco
Strawberries	Currants: red,	Salad leaves	Damsons	Sloes	broccoli
Watercress	white, black	Sorrel	Dill	Sorrel	Rosemary
Wild garlic	Dill	Spinach	Elderberries	Squash	Salsify (oyster
(ramps)	Elderflowers	Spring onions	Fennel	Swedes	plant)
	Fennel	(scallions)	(finocchio)	(rutabagas)	Shallots
	(finocchio)	Squash	Field mushrooms	Sweetcorn	Squash
	Figs	Strawberries	Figs	Tarragon	Swedes
	Fresh peas	Summer savory	Grapes	Tatsoi	(rutabagas)
	Garlic	Sweetcorn	Horseradish	Thyme	Turnips
	Globe artichokes	Tarragon	Jerusalem	Turnips	Winter savory
	Gooseberries	Thyme	artichokes	Watercress	
	Green beans	Tomatoes	Kale	Winter savory	
	Greengages	Turnips	Kohlrabi		
	Jerusalem	Watercress	Lavender		
	artichoke				
	Kohlrabi				

THE POWER OF VARIETY

Read almost any magazine article or government recommendation on the topic of diet and you're likely to read: 'Eat a variety of fruit and vegetables.' A varied diet is clearly thought to be a cornerstone of healthy eating. But why? What's the big deal?

DIET PATTERNS

What's wrong with finding a few meals that you like and can cook, and being content with those? There are a couple of answers.

The first is that if you never altered your meal plans you would probably get bored. Trying new foods is a natural drive that can help you to maintain interest in your diet. It's a pleasure to browse recipes and to find new favourites; eating new foods creates anticipation, which actually gets your digestive juices going.

In between these extremes – the boredom of an unchanging diet and the thrill of discovering new foods – is your 'usual' way of eating. The term currently in use is your 'diet pattern' – the set of habits that shape your personal way of eating. Daily reliance on processed and junk foods, or a habit of constant snacking throughout the day are diet-pattern disasters. It takes only two or three days for one of these to become your adopted diet pattern. It will take a little longer – but perhaps only a few weeks – for it to become a full-blown pattern of malnutrition. Variety can break that pattern to save the day, your waistline and possibly your health.

There is a second reason why variety in your diet is encouraged. Simply, you are much more likely to obtain all the nutrients you need when you eat a varied diet. Nutrients not found in one food might be abundant in another. When you bring these natural differences together in one diet pattern, you fill the gaps in your nutrition. Any nutritional deficiencies that have arisen (and which can be the cause of chronic disease or disorders) can be resolved. Variety, in your fruit and vegetable intake especially, is likely to reduce your risk of heart disease and may protect you against some types of cancer, as well as providing sufficient nutrients for all your needs. When you create sufficiency, you can enjoy good health.

UPGRADE YOUR PATTERNS

Building variety into your diet is not difficult. You will need to give your attention to it for just a few days – after that it takes very little effort because it becomes a positive, supportive habit. Following the key ideas of eating whole, local and seasonal will naturally bring variety to your diet.

When the season for a particular food passes, simply move on to the foods that are newly arrived on the market. This is nature's way of offering variety.

FINE-TUNE YOUR APPROACH

Seek out one of the vegan food group charts or pyramids. These have six to twelve food groups including, for instance: fruit, root or starchy vegetables; green vegetables; orange and red vegetables; beans and lentils; nuts and seeds; whole grains; fats and oils; mushrooms and yeast products; sea vegetables; and plant-based beverages. The idea is to eat across these groups to help you to build variety into your diet.

Choosing the number of servings to be eaten from each category of plant foods is another approach. For instance, the US government recommends five to thirteen portions of fruit and vegetables daily; the UK government suggests five. These are broad guidelines combining two or more food groups, but they do underline the fact that variety is necessary if you intend to meet those numbers (few of us would want to eat thirteen bananas per day!).

Intake of macronutrients (fat, protein, carbohydrate) is sometimes measured as a percentage of calories. This approach to variety won't suit everyone, but it can provide a framework for your food choices. For instance, the World Health Organization recommends less than 30 per cent of daily calorie intake from all fats, with saturated fats reduced to no more than 10 per cent and an urgent elimination of all manufactured trans fats (trans-fatty acids). Similar recommendations are provided by most governments and health advisory services.

Recent nutrition projects use colour coding to help people to build variety into their diets. Plant foods are grouped according to pigmentation – foods with similar colouring have been shown to have phytochemical qualities in common. The advice is to eat from each of five colour categories (red, orange/yellow, green, blue/purple and white), to derive a wide variety of phytochemicals from your diet.

PLATES AND PICTURES

An approach that neatly combines all of these suggestions is one that was presented in a lecture given by Michael Klaper, MD, at the Royal Homoeopathic Hospital in London. He suggested a template for how a plate of healthy food should be apportioned, likening the picture it creates to a 'cartoon mouse of some fame':

* Half of the plate should provide energy-rich starchy carbohydrates, such as grains or potatoes.
* One quarter should comprise green vegetables.
* One quarter should be yellow/orange vegetables.
* One 'ear' should be a serving of protein-rich foods such as beans, nuts or seeds.
* The other 'ear' should be fruit, preferably those that are coloured blue/purple, red or yellow/orange.

The 'plate' approach is a very popular one now and various versions of it exist. It is highly visual, easy to achieve and naturally can include a great range of nutrients from a variety of foods.

GEAR FOR A VEGAN KITCHEN

You can switch to a vegan diet using the basic utensils you might already have in a family kitchen: knives, a chopping board, a sieve and colander, a mixing bowl, a pan or two, and a wooden spoon and spatula. If you are replacing items or just setting up a kitchen, these suggestions can help you to invest wisely:

* Pans ideally should be cast iron, enamel or stainless steel. If you intend to purchase new pans, go for simplicity and buy those that will last the longest.
* Nonstick finishes are not necessary.
* Oven-to-table dishes that have lids are versatile and practical.
* A set of glass mixing bowls is always useful.
* A vegetable steamer lets you preserve nutrients, flavour and texture in cooked vegetables. Steamers are available as stacked units over a saucepan, allowing you to steam different vegetables at once, or as adjustable 'baskets' that expand or contract to fit most pan sizes.

Certain implements ease the preparation of the meals you are likely to prepare. For instance:

* Salad spinner: used to spin-dry rinsed leaves; also stores them well in the refrigerator
* Pressure cooker: very time- and energy-efficient; used predominantly for beans
* Mouli (rotary food mill): for sauces, jams (jellies) and chutneys, soups and some bean dishes
* Hand-held blender 'wand': to make smoothies, soups, sauces and some batters
* Kitchen scales, measuring spoons and a measuring jug (large measuring cup): to help to get proportions right

Small items can be collected over time. Some can make a difference to how quick and easy it is for you to make favourite dishes:

* Mortar and pestle: for grinding spice mixtures and flaxseed (linseed) from fresh
* Silicon garlic peeler: insert the garlic clove, roll the silicon tube and … it works!
* Garlic press: to make crushed garlic for your salad dressings
* Ginger grater: hand-held and uses tiny spikes rather than blades
* Nut grinder (nut mill): a small hand-turned mill that catches all the nutty bits
* Lemon or citrus press: to squeeze out the juice
* Olive-pit remover: pushes the pit out when you squeeze the device

Speciality tools are fun to have, especially if you become an expert in a dish or style of cooking, but are not needed for any of the recipes in this book. If there is something that really appeals, add it to your birthday wish list and see what happens.

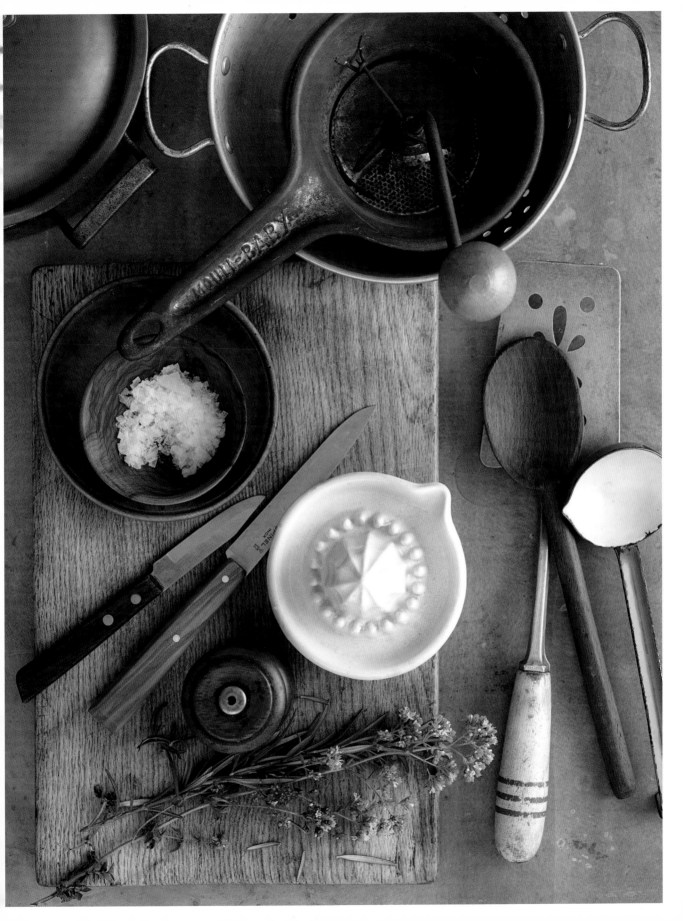

NUTRITION 101

This chart outlines a basic framework of nutrition that will guide you toward eating a healthy diet. Essential nutrients are divided into two categories: macronutrients and micronutrients. The four macronutrients are required in fairly large amounts on a daily basis. There are two subcategories of micronutrients – vitamins and minerals – and minerals are divided into macroelements and microelements. Macroelements are required at a level of 100 milligrams (mg) per day or more, while microelements are required at levels of a few milligrams or less. With the possible exception of cobalt, all these nutrients are amply provided by a varied diet of whole grains, greens, beans and lentils, vegetables, nuts, yeast products and sea vegetables.

NUTRIENT	BENEFIT	SOURCE
MACRONUTRIENTS		
CARBOHYDRATES	Provide a major source of fuel for the body; contain vitamins, minerals, proteins, fats and water. Simple carbohydrates provide 'instant' energy. Complex carbohydrates provide slow-release energy and fibre	Simple carbohydrates from sugars; complex carbohydrates from whole or unrefined plant foods such as whole grains, pulses, fruit and vegetables
PROTEINS	Often called the 'building blocks of life'; build, maintain and repair body tissues; instigate and control cellular processes	Every plant and every thing living or that once was alive
FATS	Required for cell function, to form hormones, to protect and enable nerve impulses and to transport vitamins	Nuts and seeds, their oils and butters, soya beans, corn, avocados
WATER	Enables transportation of vitamins, minerals and other nutrients; helps to regulate body temperature and enables excretion through urine, perspiration and breath; lubricates bowels, joints and mucus lining of the airways	Fruits, vegetables, plant milks, herbal teas, juices, fresh water
MICRONUTRIENTS		
VITAMINS		
VITAMIN D	Assists in absorption of minerals crucial to bone health and kidney function	Daily 30-minute exposure of skin to daylight
VITAMIN A	Influences normal growth, preserves night vision and aids in the normal development of bones and teeth	Green and yellow vegetables, yellow and orange fruits, nuts, seeds and whole grains
VITAMIN E	An antioxidant, important to reproductive health and manufacture of hormonelike prostaglandins	
VITAMIN K	Can be manufactured in the intestinal tract; helps normal blood-clotting	
VITAMIN C (ASCORBIC ACID)	Strengthens capillary walls, helps wounds to heal, helps to resolve allergic and immune responses; can boost your absorption of non-haem iron	Citrus fruits, melons, tomatoes, peppers (capsicums), leafy greens, cabbage, potato with its peel
VITAMIN B GROUP	Aid digestion; reduce stress; benefit skin, hair, nails, nerves and eyes; and are involved in growth, immunity and metabolism	Whole grains, leafy greens, beans and lentils, potatoes, yellow vegetables, dried fruits, nuts, yeast products, mushrooms and molasses

NUTRIENT	BENEFIT	SOURCE
MINERALS (MACROELEMENTS)		
CALCIUM	Influences bone structure, nerve impulses, muscle contractions, metabolism and the action of many hormones, enzymes and cell activities	Broccoli, cabbage, green leafy vegetables, nuts and seeds, pulses
CHLORIDE	Works with sodium to control fluid outside the cell membrane	Sea salt
MAGNESIUM	Influences mineral balance, bone development, protein manufacture, muscle contraction and release, nerve impulses and actions of B vitamins	Green leafy vegetables, nuts and seeds, whole grains, soya beans, dark chocolate
PHOSPHORUS	Helps to metabolize fats and carbohydrates, promotes healthy nerves, growth and repair, and strengthens bones and teeth	Soya beans, nuts, whole grains, yeast products
POTASSIUM	Regulates fluid inside the cell membrane; stimulates stomach and pancreatic secretions	Dried fruits, bananas, avocados, tomatoes, nuts, potatoes, salad greens, molasses
SODIUM	Works with potassium to maintain fluid movement through cells; aids nerve impulses	Fresh fruits and vegetables, peas, celery, sea salt
SULPHUR	Aids in the production of collagen; benefits skin, hair and nails; combats autoimmune disorders	Nuts, garlic, beans, radishes, watercress
MINERALS (MICROELEMENTS)		
CHROMIUM	Influential in regulating blood sugar and may promote cardiovascular health	Peanuts, grape juice, black pepper, beans, potatoes, carrots, apples
COBALT	Required for the formation of vitamin B_{12} molecule	Vitamin B_{12}
COPPER	Aids absorption of iron, regulation of cholesterol, health of nerves	Almonds, walnuts, sunflower seeds, Brazil nuts, mushrooms
FLUORIDE	Said to strengthen teeth and bones	Sea salt, potatoes, tea
IODINE	Increases energy, improves immunity, improves mental function	Sunflower seeds, seaweed, mushrooms
IRON	Transports oxygen to body cells and carbon dioxide to the lungs for excretion	Raisins, red wine, beans, peanut butter, molasses
MANGANESE	Important in the production of hormones and in endocrine function	Beetroot (beets), nuts and seeds, grains, olives, avocados, tea
MOLYBDENUM	Protects teeth against decay, promotes enzyme activity	Green beans, sunflower seeds, lentils, soya beans, oats and peas
SELENIUM	Antioxidant that works with vitamin E; aids immunity, helps to prevent degenerative diseases	Brazil nuts, molasses, peanuts, brewer's yeast, wheat bran
ZINC	Increases immunity, soothes nerve and mental disorders, assists growth and healing of wounds, may reduce susceptibility to diabetes	Nuts and seeds, green leafy vegetables, pre-soaked whole grains and beans
PHYTOCHEMICALS	Consumption is associated with a reduction in risk of several chronic diseases and may have protective and preventive effects	Whole foods

FROM FOOD OR SUPPLEMENT?

No matter what sort of diet you eat, the following four nutrients are crucial to good health. However, each of them needs you to understand when – or if – supplementation is beneficial.

FOLATE FROM FOOD

Folate is a naturally occurring member of the B group of vitamins, also known as B_9 or folacin. Folate supports fertility in both men and women. It acts on the immune system, on the manufacture of amino acids, on cell division and on the formation of red blood cells. Folate (B_9) is made more effective by the presence of vitamin B_{12} in your diet.

For adults, 400 micrograms (mcg) of folate per day is considered sufficient and supplements are not usually recommended, provided a variety of folate-rich food is eaten on a daily basis. Folate is naturally present in many foods, but especially dark green leafy vegetables. Good sources include:

* leafy vegetables such as spinach, cabbage and cos (romaine) lettuce
* broccoli, Brussels sprouts, kale and cauliflower
* asparagus
* avocados
* okra
* lentils, peas and beans
* nuts and seeds
* fresh oranges and dates

FOLIC ACID FROM SUPPLEMENTS

There is also a manufactured (synthetic) form of folate. It is called folic acid and is used to fortify processed foods. You have probably seen this term on food labels, including:

* breads and breakfast cereals
* yeast products such as yeast extract and nutritional yeast flakes

For a healthy adult, folic acid intake from supplements and fortified foods should not exceed 1000mcg per day, as great amounts of it can mask symptoms of vitamin B_{12} deficiency. The measurement of both folate and folic acid is given in micrograms, abbreviated to mcg or µg. There are 1000mcg in a milligram (mg), and 1000mg in a gram (g).

In pregnancy, folate helps to reduce the risk of your child suffering a neural tube defect such as spina bifida. These generally occur in early pregnancy, so you are advised to optimize your intake of folate before you become pregnant. A vegan diet is naturally abundant in folate. However, to allay concerns, current medical guidance is that women who are planning a pregnancy should take 400mcg daily of a folic acid supplement prior to stopping contraception and then for the first twelve weeks of the pregnancy. Please discuss this guidance with your doctor or midwife, as it is possible to take too much folic acid, the manufactured form of folate.

YOUR CHOICE

You will be reassured to know that 400mcg of folate is easy to acquire from your food, especially for a person eating a varied vegan diet. A small side dish of cooked spinach (100g/3½oz/½ cup), for instance, can provide one quarter of the recommended amount. Salads, greens, lentils, fruit, and nuts or seeds eaten during the course of a day are likely to complete the recommended amount comfortably. Any fortified foods you eat will then supplement this natural intake.

VITAMIN B12 FROM FOOD

B_{12} is necessary for healthy neurological function, the production of red blood cells, maintenance of the nervous system, nutrient assimilation, fertility, growth, immunity and DNA manufacture. Deficiency of this vitamin can lead to life-changing anaemia and damage to the nervous system. This vitamin is produced by bacteria and absorbed by way of an enzyme in your gastric juices. Shortage of this enzyme can be brought about by ageing, illness or surgery. That and continuing uncertainty as to the sources and availability of B_{12} make this a controversial and sometimes bewildering nutrient.

Plant foods reported as being sources of B_{12} include shiitake mushrooms, dried nori seaweed and fermented bean or vegetable products such as miso, kimchi, sauerkraut and pickles. However, this is where uncertainty lies: the amounts present may be trace levels or in biologically unavailable forms.

FROM SUPPLEMENTS

Medical guidance cautions that vitamin B_{12} is not provided in the vegan diet except by fortification or supplementation.

* The US National Institutes of Health currently states that vitamin B_{12} 'is generally not present in plant foods', but points out that fortified foods are available.
* The Vegan Society, in cooperation with the International Vegetarian Union Science Group, produced a document on B_{12} in which it recommends that this nutrient be taken in adequate amounts through the use of fortified foods or supplements.
* Supplements are made in a laboratory without the use of any animal product and are available in tablet, capsule, liquid or gel form.
* Foods such as yeast extract, nutritional yeast flakes, some plant milks and many breads and breakfast cereals are fortified with B_{12}; please check the labels.

* Vitamin B_{12} is required in minute amounts, measured in micrograms (mcg or μg). You need approximately 1.5mcg per day to maintain health. However, only about half of what you take in through your food or in supplements will be absorbed.
* The recommended intake for adults is set at 2.4–3mcg per day, to allow for 50 per cent absorption.
* Slightly more is recommended during pregnancy and lactation – 2.6 and 2.8mcg, respectively.
* Adults over 50 years of age sometimes are advised to take more than these amounts.

Your body can absorb only tiny amounts of B_{12} at any given time, so small but frequent doses are best. Although you may retain stores of B_{12} in your liver and kidneys, it is a water-soluble vitamin and any excess is excreted in your urine. Combine or alternate these options to provide sufficient B_{12}:

* Take 3mcg per day, in 1mcg doses, three times during the day.
* Take at least 10mcg per day if you take only one dose during the day.
* Take a large dose of approximately 2000mcg, once a week.

YOUR CHOICE

Vitamin B_{12} deficiency can be experienced by omnivores, vegetarians and vegans alike. For your long-term health, and to act responsibly for yourself and your loved ones, please ensure that you include a supplement or fortified foods in your diet.

IRON FROM FOOD

Iron is a trace mineral essential to human health. Your body will contain 3–4mg of iron, most of it in the form of haemoglobin, the red pigment in your blood that transports oxygen to your cells. Iron is also present in myoglobin, in muscles; it is recycled in the spleen and stored in bone marrow and the liver. Like so many nutrients, iron works best in conjunction with other minerals and vitamins, including folate and vitamin B_{12} (see pages 22–4). For this reason, it is best to derive it from a wide variety of whole foods. Plant foods rich in iron include:

* dark green leafy vegetables
* dried fruit such as raisins, figs and apricots
* nuts and seeds
* lentils and beans
* whole grains
* molasses
* seaweed
* dark chocolate

Plant foods contain only non-haem iron; animal flesh contains about 60 per cent non-haem iron and 40 per cent haem iron. The non-haem iron from either source is less readily absorbed than haem iron, possibly to ensure that iron intake is not excessive. Your body's absorption of non-haem iron is increased when you eat foods high in vitamin C during the same meal. It is easy to prepare vegan meals that include both iron-rich and vitamin C-rich food, such as fruits, sweet peppers (capsicums), cauliflower, green leafy vegetables, cabbage and tomatoes.

The recommended daily allowance (RDA) for an adult male is 8mg; for an adult female of childbearing age it is 18mg, reducing to 8mg for women over 50 years of age. Iron requirements in pregnancy are higher, at 27mg, to provide for an increase in blood volume in the mother and to put in place an adequate store of iron in the infant's liver. This store ensures the infant has a supply of iron during their early months when feeding solely on breast milk, which naturally contains very little iron.

IRON FROM SUPPLEMENTS

Many processed foods, such as breakfast cereals, are fortified with iron. As well, there are a great many iron supplements available on the market. However, current medical guidance cautions against taking high doses (more than 15–17mg per day) of supplemental iron and suggests that most people should be able to meet their iron requirements through a varied diet.

YOUR CHOICE

Your body naturally conserves and recycles iron, whatever its source. If you are deficient, your body tries to increase the amount it absorbs from your diet. You lose some iron each day through your stool and as your skin replenishes. However, your body has no mechanism for excreting excess iron except by bleeding. This is why excess iron intake can create serious health problems and why upper limits are set for supplementation. Absorption of iron is inhibited by obesity and enhanced by variety in the diet.

CALCIUM FROM FOOD

Most of the calcium in your body is in your teeth and bones. A small amount circulates in your blood and is used for healthy nerve function, the action of enzymes, muscle contraction and numerous cell activities. Meanwhile, your bones are constantly being remodelled in a process that requires the movement of not only calcium, but magnesium and phosphorus, too.

Current guidance suggests both men and women maintain an intake of 700–1000mg calcium per day, taken *through their diet*. Young people and the elderly might require more, up to 1200mg per day.

Ensuring you have enough calcium in your diet is especially important for pregnant women, as it decreases the risk of complications such as pre-eclampsia. If you hope to get pregnant, sort out your calcium intake now so that you feel confident you will be building good bones for your child. Simple changes and inclusions to your diet will make this pleasing and easy to achieve, even into the period of lactation.

Actual daily intake of calcium varies significantly by region, with Scandinavian, northern European and other non-equatorial areas consuming the most. Ideal intakes are rarely achieved except in northern regions. The difference between recommended and actual intake raises questions when one sees that rates of osteoporosis and osteopenia are often higher in populations with a high intake of calcium.

Some feel this is due to too much emphasis being placed on calcium alone when, in fact, calcium metabolism requires magnesium, phosphorus, vitamin D and other nutrient companions. It seems prudent to include mineral-rich foods in your diet and to take regular weight-bearing exercise outdoors. Thirty minutes of sunlight is needed each day to make vitamin D, which helps you to absorb the minerals in your food and maintain bone health.

Whether you are male or female, it is easy to derive 1000mg of calcium from what you eat and drink each day. If you live in a 'hard' water area, your drinking water can provide up to 500mg of your calcium needs each day. Plant foods rich in calcium, magnesium and phosphorus include:

* dark green leafy vegetables such as kale, cabbage, chard (silver beet), parsley and watercress
* beans and lentils
* whole grains
* dried fruits
* nuts and seeds
* molasses
* seaweed
* dark chocolate

CALCIUM FROM SUPPLEMENTS

Side effects from calcium supplementation can include constipation, kidney stones and, in some, an increased risk of heart attack. These are unlikely when calcium is derived from the diet or from occasional use of calcium-fortified foods.

YOUR CHOICE

Please discuss taking a supplement with your doctor or midwife if you feel you cannot align your diet to meet a healthy intake of calcium each day. It is very difficult to take too much calcium through your diet, but be aware that calcium supplements can cause unpleasant side effects, especially if, in your enthusiasm, you take too much.

THE PROTEIN QUESTION

A common question asked of vegans is: 'Where do you get your protein?'

It's reasonable enough, given that so many people equate protein with meat. Yes, it's true that muscle tissue is protein-rich (so, too, are hair, skin, nails, claws and horn). But protein itself is abundant in nature and takes many forms.

Every living thing, and everything that was once alive, contains protein. Proteins are made up of chains of amino acids and contain carbon, hydrogen, oxygen and, crucially, nitrogen. Plants make protein using nitrogen either from the soil or from bacteria living on their roots. Protein is present in all plants.

In our bodies, proteins build, repair and maintain tissues. They also can be a source of energy and form hormones, vitamins and enzymes. As enzymes, proteins are involved in many metabolic processes. Proteins instigate and control most cellular activities. They influence the immune system, take part in the transport of vitamins, minerals and fatty acids, and are present in various body fluids.

Currently, twenty amino acids are recognized as being present in most proteins. Ten of these are found in body tissues; a further nine are necessary but must be obtained from your diet. These necessary amino acids are called 'indispensable' or 'essential' amino acids. The importance placed on variety in your diet is partly to ensure that all of these essential amino acids are acquired on a regular basis because each one has a specific influence within the body.

Requirements for protein vary from person to person and are influenced by age, gender, level of activity and general state of health. Various regional and global recommendations currently give guidance that, for adults, protein should comprise 10–12 per cent of calorie intake. This equates to approximately 0.8g of protein per kilogram of body weight. Recommendations for children are higher per kilogram of body weight because children are growing rapidly. We need protein in combination with other nutrients; that's what whole foods do for us.

* Protein is available from all plant-based foods. Protein-rich plant foods include microalgae, yeast products, sea vegetables, soya beans, their products and all the beans and pulses, nuts, seeds, whole grains, vegetables and fruit.
* Many of the pulses have a 'percentage of calories as protein' that is higher than meat. Soya beans, for example, provide 40 per cent of their calorie value as protein.
* Protein intake is normally adequate if calorie needs are met from a variety of whole foods.
* Combining foods to create 'complete proteins' in each meal is no longer considered necessary, provided you eat from a variety of whole foods.

Next time you are asked the protein question, you can answer: 'Protein is everywhere! I eat a wide selection of whole, plant-based foods and they give me all I need.'

COOKING SAVVY

Recipes are wonderful inventions, but don't let them stifle your 'inner cook'. Preparing a dish should be your unique response to the ingredients you have to hand. A recipe can guide you with precise instructions or it can give you a broad idea of what to do and how the dish might turn out. But the most important ingredient is you.

Cooking starts with you, a work surface laden with fresh goods and the questions that pop into your mind. What is this? You pick it up. What does it smell like? You hold it to your nose. Is it fresh? You feel its weight and firmness. How does it grow? You study the obvious signs. But perhaps you don't know. Perhaps you have always lived in town, never had a garden, never gone on a 'pick your own' excursion. Now is your chance to get some savvy.

USE YOUR HANDS

Many people under the age of 50 have only ever bought food in a packaged or pretreated form. The production of food has been relegated to others, usually far away from our locale. We pay the prices because we are liberated from the work – but we are also deprived of an authentic experience of what food really is. There is a cycle of growth, harvesting, storage and waste that our recent ancestors knew very well, but about which we might have no knowledge. This is a disconnect with profound implications.

Currently, just over half (55 per cent) of the world's population live in cities. Urban design limits the number of households that have any outdoor space, but particularly space that includes a patch of soil. The United Nations estimates that by 2050 the number of people living in cities will be 68 per cent of the world's population. Unless they are fortunate and have a little growing space, these people will be totally reliant on food producers to supply them – and totally reliant on whatever they are supplied.

Many food products sold today are simulacra of real food. They might have one recognizable food ingredient, but the rest on the list are names of chemicals. They might have the appearance of an old-fashioned staple, but are nearly devoid of nutrients, with substances added to extend, preserve, colour, flavour, fortify or otherwise boost the commercial value of the product. Most of us have little knowledge of and no control over these inclusions. (Some brave souls work to minimize or prevent 'fake food', especially on a corporate scale. If you ever meet one of them, thank them.)

In the meantime, you can begin to rewire the disconnect by using your hands. Eat with your hands, like a child might, or set out 'finger foods' for grown-up friends. Sprinkle salt, knead dough, shape patties and arrange a salad. Using your hands alerts you to qualities and characteristics that cannot be labelled. Hands are delicate antennae that pat shoulders, beat applause and clasp hold of another. Use yours, as well, to reclaim your connection with the life forms that sustain you.

MANY HANDS MAKE LIGHT WORK

Children need to learn about and connect with food, too. Keep children out of the kitchen and you will keep them in unskilled ignorance until young adulthood or beyond. Share cooking with them now and you'll create skill and some wonderful moments and memories.

Open the kitchen doors and let the party begin! The tasks and roles you give them must be genuinely helpful because you can't fool them – they will know if you are fobbing them off with 'kiddie' work. They must be true participants, making valuable contributions. A bit of chaos naturally ensues when people cluster together to do a job. Let it go! You can clean up any mess and do things your way again – later. Right now, roll up your sleeves and get happy. Making a meal happens in four stages:

* **PLANNING** Decide what you want to make, gather the ingredients and think about timings so that everything is ready when you need it.
* **PREPARING** Share out the many small tasks and get everyone busy. At first, this will seem like ten times the effort – and it probably *is* ten times the effort the first few times – but stay relaxed. It's worth it.
* **SERVING** If the project gets this far it is a success! Do a group review of the meal while you are eating it and arrange another date to do it all again.
* **FOLLOW THROUGH** Clear the table, wash up and put everything away. No one wants to do this part, but it goes really quickly if everyone pitches in to help.

Necessary tasks that are also social usually bring out the best in people. In a cooperative effort, the boundaries between people can seem less significant. As well, there is much to talk about. For instance, how do you grate a carrot without losing your fingernails? How do you not cry when peeling an onion? Do Australians stir the pot counterclockwise? Does the alphabet soup have all the letters of the alphabet?

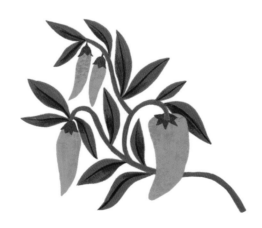

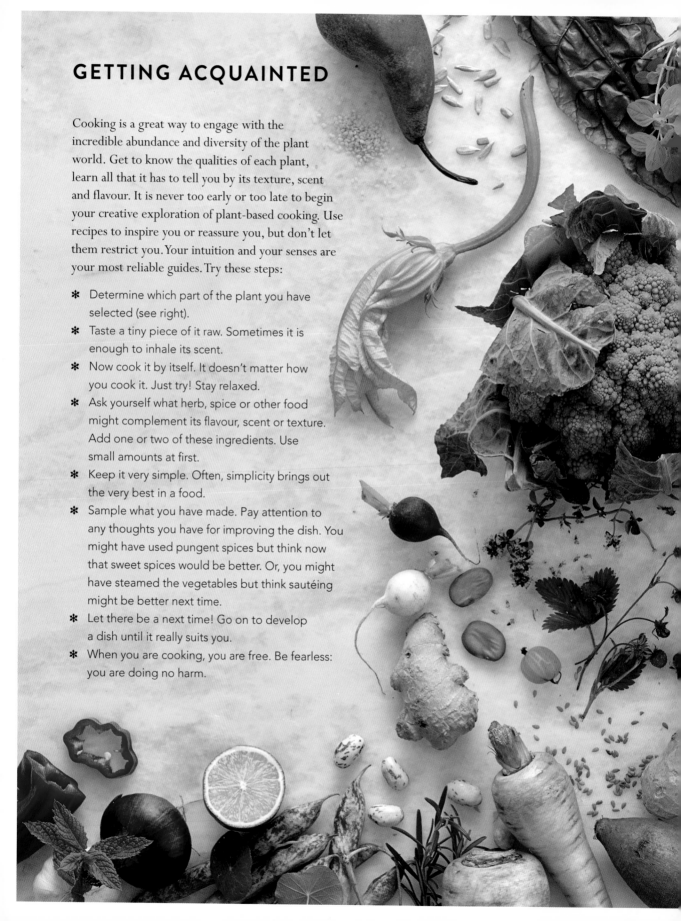

GETTING ACQUAINTED

Cooking is a great way to engage with the incredible abundance and diversity of the plant world. Get to know the qualities of each plant, learn all that it has to tell you by its texture, scent and flavour. It is never too early or too late to begin your creative exploration of plant-based cooking. Use recipes to inspire you or reassure you, but don't let them restrict you. Your intuition and your senses are your most reliable guides. Try these steps:

* Determine which part of the plant you have selected (see right).
* Taste a tiny piece of it raw. Sometimes it is enough to inhale its scent.
* Now cook it by itself. It doesn't matter how you cook it. Just try! Stay relaxed.
* Ask yourself what herb, spice or other food might complement its flavour, scent or texture. Add one or two of these ingredients. Use small amounts at first.
* Keep it very simple. Often, simplicity brings out the very best in a food.
* Sample what you have made. Pay attention to any thoughts you have for improving the dish. You might have used pungent spices but think now that sweet spices would be better. Or, you might have steamed the vegetables but think sautéing might be better next time.
* Let there be a next time! Go on to develop a dish until it really suits you.
* When you are cooking, you are free. Be fearless: you are doing no harm.

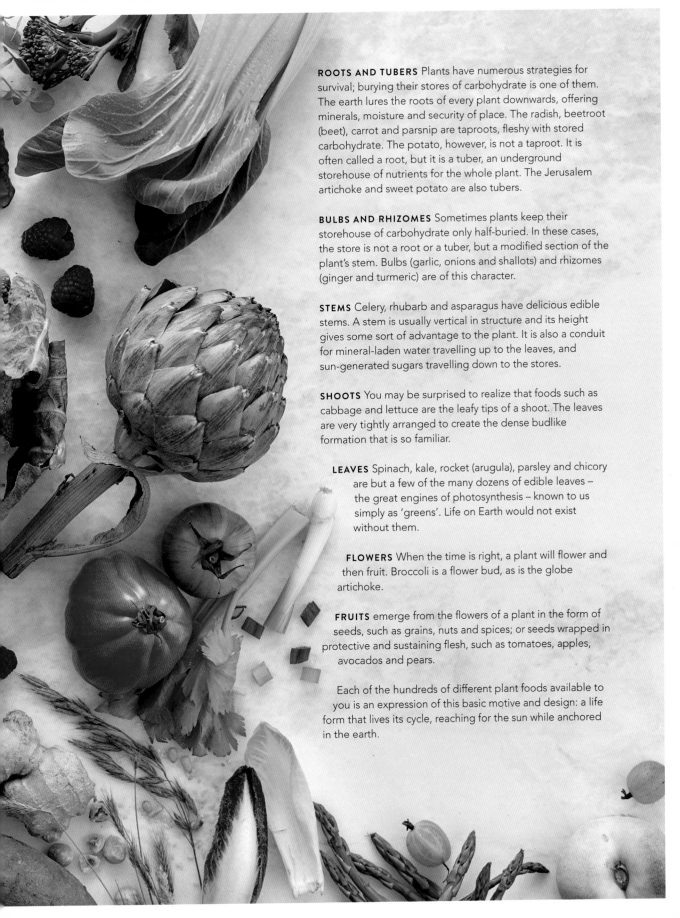

ROOTS AND TUBERS Plants have numerous strategies for survival; burying their stores of carbohydrate is one of them. The earth lures the roots of every plant downwards, offering minerals, moisture and security of place. The radish, beetroot (beet), carrot and parsnip are taproots, fleshy with stored carbohydrate. The potato, however, is not a taproot. It is often called a root, but it is a tuber, an underground storehouse of nutrients for the whole plant. The Jerusalem artichoke and sweet potato are also tubers.

BULBS AND RHIZOMES Sometimes plants keep their storehouse of carbohydrate only half-buried. In these cases, the store is not a root or a tuber, but a modified section of the plant's stem. Bulbs (garlic, onions and shallots) and rhizomes (ginger and turmeric) are of this character.

STEMS Celery, rhubarb and asparagus have delicious edible stems. A stem is usually vertical in structure and its height gives some sort of advantage to the plant. It is also a conduit for mineral-laden water travelling up to the leaves, and sun-generated sugars travelling down to the stores.

SHOOTS You may be surprised to realize that foods such as cabbage and lettuce are the leafy tips of a shoot. The leaves are very tightly arranged to create the dense budlike formation that is so familiar.

LEAVES Spinach, kale, rocket (arugula), parsley and chicory are but a few of the many dozens of edible leaves – the great engines of photosynthesis – known to us simply as 'greens'. Life on Earth would not exist without them.

FLOWERS When the time is right, a plant will flower and then fruit. Broccoli is a flower bud, as is the globe artichoke.

FRUITS emerge from the flowers of a plant in the form of seeds, such as grains, nuts and spices; or seeds wrapped in protective and sustaining flesh, such as tomatoes, apples, avocados and pears.

Each of the hundreds of different plant foods available to you is an expression of this basic motive and design: a life form that lives its cycle, reaching for the sun while anchored in the earth.

LET TIME DO THE WORK

Time achieves a great deal all by itself, when you let it. Here are four of the most satisfying but time-consuming culinary projects and how to make them fit calmly and easily into your life.

BEANS All those colourful and exotic beans from around the world are cheaper and easier to get hold of in their dried form. Before you cook them, dried beans need to be soaked in cold water for 8–24 hours. But don't panic. Putting them to soak takes less than 5 minutes. Then follow the steps in How to Cook Beans on page 64. Using only 15 minutes of your dedicated time you can have nearly a week's supply of plump, tender beans to use in any way you like.

BREADS A similar idea applies to bread-making. All you have to do is be around at the start, briefly in the middle and while the loaves are cooking. Here is what you do:

* Pick a recipe and prepare the dough. This phase includes kneading the dough – an essential step that should never be rushed. You can prepare and knead the dough in about 15 minutes. Next, cover the dough and go do something else.
* Some time later (how much later depends on the recipe but generally 2 hours), knead the dough for 2 minutes, shape it into loaves, place these in bread pans or on a baking stone, and leave them to rise again for 1–2 hours.
* Bake the raised loaves in a preheated oven. All you have to do is put them in the oven and, half an hour later, take them out!

MARINADES This method is the ultimate in letting time be your 'personal assistant':

* Select a recipe for a marinade. These are usually very quick to make because they are all combinations of flavours (such as garlic or onion, spices or herbs).
* Choose a carrier that is usually slightly acidic (such as vinegar, orange, lemon or lime juice, wine or apple juice).
* Immerse the vegetables, tofu or tempeh in the marinade.
* Cover, let it marinate for up to 24 hours, then serve!

FLAVOUR BLENDING In this method, you prepare or cook the dish, then leave it covered, usually in the refrigerator, for 4–24 hours. During this time, the flavours blend and develop, often significantly, and always for the better.

* Most soups will benefit from letting the flavours mature for a period of time.
* Vegetable pies, lasagne and many sauces can also improve from 'standing'.
* Some salads, such as bean salads and the chopped or grated salads, improve if they are covered and stored in the refrigerator for a short while (1–4 hours) before serving.

It's a matter of thinking ahead. Time prepares these foods for you, in the background, while you do other things. Once you create a habit of planning in this way, it feels reassuring. All you have to do is get the process started.

1–2–3 GOOD MORNING

Adopting these simple habits each morning will help you – and your children – to improve mood, mental focus, attention span and motivation.

1 Drink a large glass of water immediately on waking. After a long sleep, it is important to replace the water lost through breathing and perspiration. This will gently kick-start body functions, including alertness, and promote regularity in bowel movements.

2 Get up a few minutes early to create a homey, loving atmosphere in the kitchen. A head start of 30 minutes might be difficult for a week or so, but you will end up loving it. (Besides, you get to use the bathroom first!) Here are some tips:

* Use half the lighting you would usually use in the kitchen.
* Put on some sound: the radio, an audio book, calm music … but, not the TV.
* Make coffee or tea for yourself first, then breakfast for you and your family.

3 See that you and your children start the day with some breakfast, however small. Not everyone is a morning person and some prefer not to breakfast at all, but a little bite now will provide big rewards later. These include:

* The brain needs fuel immediately after sleep, which is essentially a long fast. Adults and especially children require foods rich in complex carbohydrates to supply 'brain food' at this time.
* No-breakfast people tend to display alarming signs as the morning moves toward noon. Grumpy, sleepy, fidgety and defocused … Not much work gets done and what does isn't very high-quality. That's what your children go through, too, if they go to school without breakfast.
* A recent study shows that children who leave home having had a healthy breakfast achieve greater academic success and have better levels of calm attention.
* People who skip breakfast are more likely to become overweight or obese. Avoidance of breakfast creates a 'nocturnal lifestyle pattern' that includes late-night eating, snacking on junk food and little physical exercise. This pattern can promote spikes in blood sugar levels and a greater risk of developing metabolic syndrome, increasing risk of stroke, heart disease and diabetes.
* Eating a healthy breakfast puts you in line with the natural light and dark cycles of the day. These affect your health and sense of well-being because they influence hormonal and metabolic processes in your body. When you establish a 'morning lifestyle pattern' you wake early with a definite interest in life – and breakfast! All of your body systems function best when you live in sync with these natural patterns.
* If you are a parent who skips breakfast, your children will notice and are more likely to become breakfast avoiders themselves.
* Finally, skipping breakfast devalues it when, in fact, it may be the most important meal of the day. Try it for a month, for you and your family, and see for yourself.

BREAKFASTS

CORN AND CARROT MUFFINS

The flavour of these muffins is a little sweet and a little earthy, thanks to the cornmeal. They're perfect in a packed lunch or for a light breakfast, with a smoothie or a cup of coffee. Serve them warm with a portion of Apple Butter (page 43), Plum Butter (page 45) or more marmalade if you want a sweeter treat – or with Scrambled Tofu (page 39) if you're in the mood for something savoury.

MAKES 12 LARGE MUFFINS

PREPARATION TIME 40 MINUTES

150g (5oz/1¼ cups) fine cornmeal

150g (5oz/1¼ cups) plain (all-purpose) or wholemeal (whole-wheat) flour

100g (3½oz/½ cup) caster (superfine) sugar

1 tablespoon baking powder

1 teaspoon ground ginger

1 medium carrot, grated

170ml (5½fl oz/⅔ cup) thin-cut marmalade

70ml (2¼fl oz) tahini

70ml (2¼fl oz) coconut oil, melted

300ml (10½fl oz/1¼ cups) plant milk

1 tablespoon apple cider vinegar

OPTIONS AND VARIATIONS

Add 1 teaspoon ground cinnamon along with the ground ginger.

Preheat the oven to 200°C (400°F), and place paper liners in a 12-hole standard muffin pan.

Mix together the cornmeal, flour, sugar, baking powder and ground ginger in a large bowl. Add the grated carrot to the dry ingredients, and stir well.

Combine the marmalade, tahini and coconut oil in a measuring jug (large measuring cup). Add the plant milk and vinegar, and stir well. Working swiftly now, tip the wet mixture into the dry ingredients and stir as briefly as possible, while ensuring that everything is thoroughly and evenly mixed.

Divide the batter evenly among the prepared paper liners. Bake for 15–20 minutes until the muffins are risen and golden, and a skewer or the tip of a sharp knife inserted into the centre of a muffin comes out clean.

Let the muffins cool a little in the pan for 5 minutes, before transferring them to a wire rack. Serve warm or cold.

✻ **FAST REACTIONS** When making vegan bakes, it's fairly common practice to add a little vinegar to the wet ingredients. Its acidity will react with the baking powder – or sometimes bicarbonate of soda (baking soda) or cream of tartar – included in the dry mix and make the cake rise. This reaction begins to happen the moment the wet ingredients make contact with the dry ingredients, so it's very important to work quickly at this stage. Getting your uncooked cake into the oven as swiftly as possible will ensure a lighter result.

ALL-SEASONS FRUIT SALAD

I like to make this luscious salad in the evening and store it in the refrigerator ready for breakfast the next day. Try some stirred into a bowl of muesli (adding more orange juice to moisten the cereal, if necessary). You can also pack it for lunch or treat yourself to a sweet, fruity dessert after dinner. As spring moves through summer and into autumn (fall), reflect the changing seasons by using different berries as they become available. Look out for mulberries, strawberries, raspberries, red, white and blackcurrants, blueberries and blackberries. You could even include a few sliced gooseberries – bearing in mind that they can be rather tart. Try varying the dried fruits, too: substitute equal quantities of chopped dried mango, prunes or pear for any of those listed.

Combine the dried fruits in a bowl and pour over the citrus juice. Add the fresh fruits and stir gently to ensure that each piece of fruit is coated with juice. Cover the dish and leave in the refrigerator to soak for at least 4 hours, but ideally all day or overnight. Stir occasionally to redistribute the juices.

❋ **THE HONEY QUESTION** Honeybees collect pollen and nectar from flowering plants, process it in their bodies, regurgitate it, concentrate it and store it in their hives. The pollen and nectar collected from approximately two million flowers is needed to make one pound of honey; it takes thousands of hours of bee work to complete the process. Many vegans refuse to include honey in their diet because they feel the bees are exploited, robbed of their store of honey and then, the final insult, not protected by humans. Globally, bees are suffering a decline in population. Most of the world's 100 most important food crops rely on bees or other pollinators; there are concerns for global food security if the bee population continues to fall. Barley malt syrup is a useful replacement for honey, but, if you decide to include honey in your diet, try to choose an organically produced one from a local beekeeper. You can promote the health of wild bees by growing plants they will visit and by growing them without chemicals. See Resources.

SERVES 4

PREPARATION TIME 15 MINUTES

+ 4 HOURS MARINATING

100g (3½oz) pitted dates, chopped (about ¾ cup prepared)

100g (3½oz) dried figs, chopped (about ⅔ cup prepared)

100g (3½oz) dried apricots, chopped (about ¾ cup prepared)

50g (1¾oz) dried goji berries (about ⅔ cup)

Juice of 2 lemons or 2 oranges (or use 1 of each)

250g (9oz) seasonal fresh berries

2 bananas, sliced

2 apples, chopped

OPTIONS AND VARIATIONS

Use 70g (2½oz/scant ½ cup) raisins instead of the goji berries. Sprinkle with sunflower seeds, or add 1 tablespoon chopped fresh mint, just before serving.

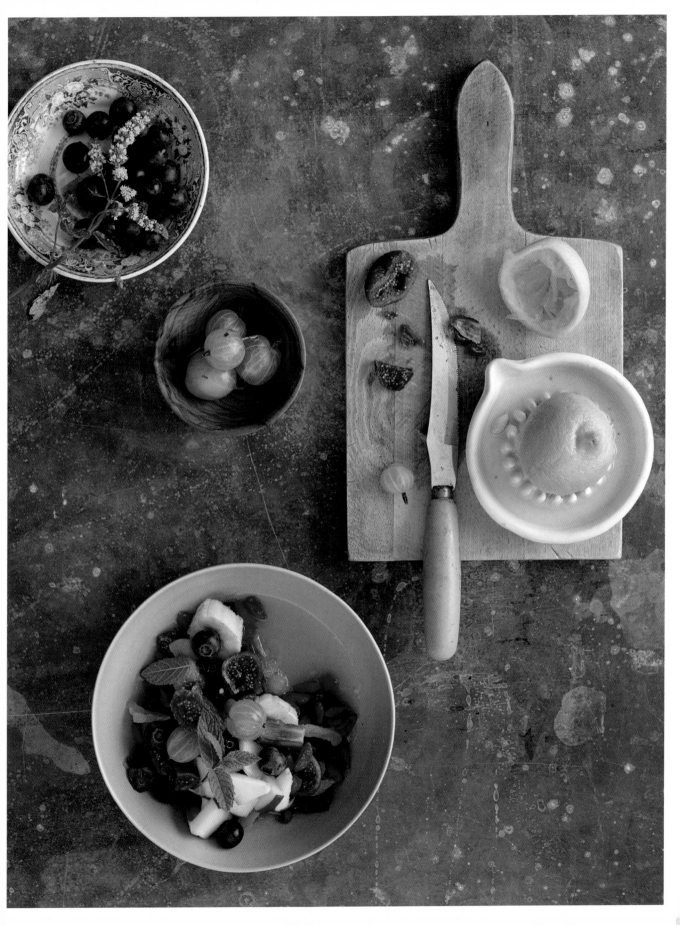

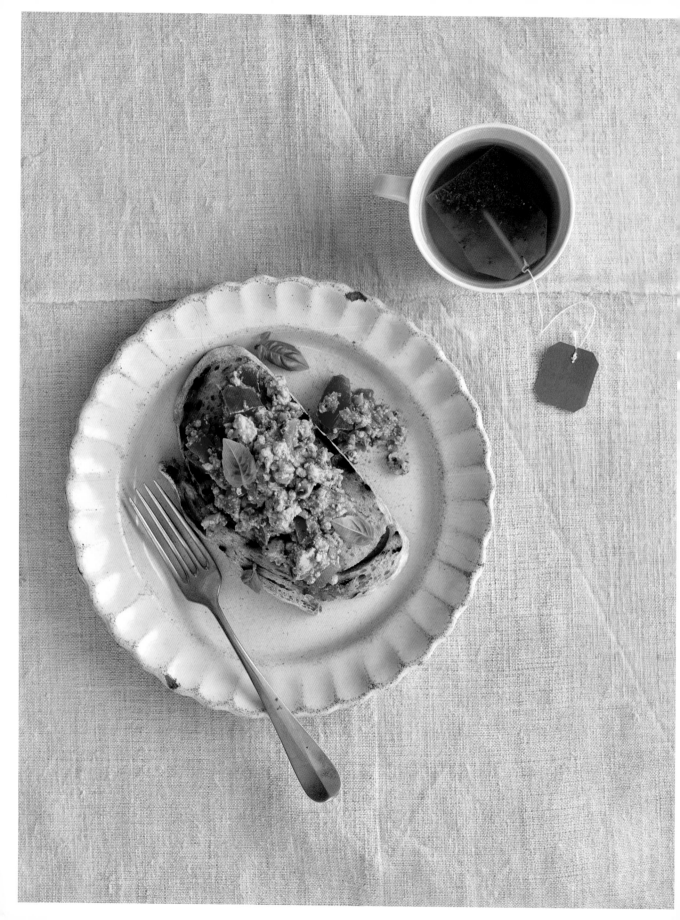

SCRAMBLED TOFU

This dish can be made to resemble scrambled eggs, or it can be treated as a tasty, vegetable-rich vegan breakfast in its own right by making a few simple additions. Either way, it's quick and easy to prepare. Serve hot over toast, as filling for a baked potato or alongside Warm Broccoli Salad (page 151).

(page 151)

SERVES 4

PREPARATION TIME 30 MINUTES

1 tablespoon untoasted sesame oil

1 small onion, finely chopped

3 garlic cloves, finely chopped

1 medium tomato, finely chopped

¼ teaspoon ground turmeric

400g (14oz) silken tofu, well drained

½ teaspoon dried basil

Salt and pepper, to taste

OPTIONS AND VARIATIONS

Try adding a selection of vegetables to this dish. To ensure quick and even cooking, cut your chosen vegetables into small pieces. Try a little diced sweet pepper (capsicum), grated carrot, or florets of purple sprouting broccoli, and fresh herbs such as parsley or wild garlic (ramps). Add them to the pan at the same time as the onion and garlic, and cook for 5 minutes. Next, add the tomato and remaining ingredients as described in the method.

Pour the oil into a saucepan set over a medium heat. Add the onion and garlic, reduce the heat, and sauté for about 5 minutes, stirring occasionally. Add the tomato, cover the pan and cook for 5 minutes. Sprinkle in the turmeric and stir well.

Crumble the tofu into the saucepan and stir well, fluffing and mashing the tofu as you do so. Cook for 5 minutes in this way, to ensure an even distribution of heat and flavours.

Stir in the basil, season with salt and pepper, and serve.

✳ **TOFU** is sold as 'soft' or 'silken' when it holds a lot of water, or 'firm' when it has had some of its water drained away. I buy all sorts and enjoy experimenting. I usually choose to press some of the water out of the silken type. Tofu is a great source of protein and can be presented in a variety of ways but, in terms of flavour, it needs your help! Unless it is one of the very firm types that has been smoked or marinated, or made with added seeds, you will find that it is bland. So, you get to jazz it up. I always try spices first, including black pepper, chilli and perhaps a little allspice. I try to keep it simple, then if something works I can build on it. Turmeric is great with tofu for two reasons: it gives it a beautiful yellow colour and it slightly thickens any sauce produced. (I have made a few mistakes with ground turmeric, such as adding so much that the dish tasted like a chalk mine – so beware!) Finally, I create 'top note' flavour and aroma by adding dried herbs in the last few minutes of cooking and perhaps a garnish of fresh herbs as I serve the dish.

SWEET POTATO PUFFS

When breakfast does not come naturally to you, but you know you are better in every way if you have a little something … here is a little something. These pastries are a bit sweet, a bit savoury, and not too big. They are lovely served with Plum Butter (page 45) or with more marmalade.

MAKES 8 PUFFS

PREPARATION TIME 1 HOUR

1 quantity Vegan Shortcrust Pastry (page 265)

300g (10½oz/2¼ cups) peeled and diced sweet potatoes

50g (1¾oz/about ¼ cup) raisins

½ teaspoon ground cinnamon

8 heaped tablespoons (about ½ cup) marmalade

OPTIONS AND VARIATIONS

For an intriguing flavour, add 4 finely chopped garlic cloves to the sweet potato mixture. You can shape the puffs any way you like, making them round or even sack-shaped.

Take the prepared pastry out of the refrigerator about 30 minutes before you need it. Preheat the oven to 200°C (400°F).

Steam the sweet potato chunks for 10–12 minutes until tender. Remove from the heat and set aside to cool.

Stir together the raisins, cinnamon and cooled sweet potato in a bowl.

Roll out the pastry to a thickness of about 5mm (¼in), and divide into eight squares. Imagining a diagonal line dividing up each pastry square, spoon a portion of sweet potato and raisin mixture on one side of that line, leaving a margin around the edge for sealing. Make a small hollow in the top of each portion of filling. Put a heaped tablespoon of marmalade into each hollow, and fold the pastry diagonally over the filling to make a triangular parcel. Line up the edges of the pastry and press together to ensure a good seal.

Bake in the oven for 10 minutes, then reduce the temperature to 180°C (350°F) and cook for another 15–20 minutes until golden.

Cool the puffs on a wire rack, and serve warm or cold.

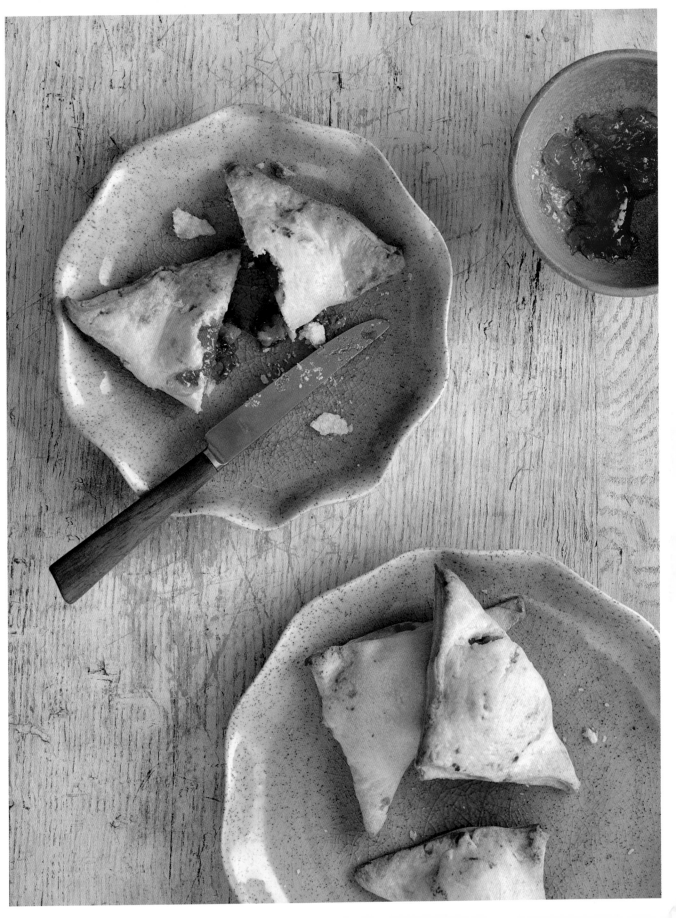

BANANA BREAD

A homey treat that is equally good for breakfast, for tea break or for a long conversation over coffee. It's not too sweet – just enough to make you wonder whether you should call it a cake. I like to serve it with berries or fresh summer fruits beside it on the plate. In winter, try a slice spread with Plum Butter (page 45).

MAKES 1 LOAF

PREPARATION TIME 1 HOUR

300g (10½oz/2⅓ cups) plain (all-purpose) or wholemeal (whole-wheat) flour

2 teaspoons baking powder

1 teaspoon ground nutmeg

½ teaspoon ground cinnamon

125g (4½oz/⅔ cup) demerara (turbinado) sugar

250ml (9fl oz/1 cup plus 2 tablespoons) plant milk

80ml (2½fl oz/⅓ cup) tahini

100g (3½oz) coconut oil, melted, plus extra for greasing the loaf pan

2 very ripe bananas, peeled and mashed

1 tablespoon apple cider vinegar

OPTIONS AND VARIATIONS

Add ½ teaspoon ground cloves along with the nutmeg and cinnamon.

Preheat the oven to 250°C (500°F), and lightly brush a 900g (2lb) loaf pan with a little melted coconut oil.

Stir the flour, baking powder and spices together in a large bowl.

In a measuring jug (large measuring cup), combine the sugar and plant milk. Stir well to dissolve the sugar, then add the tahini, whisking to make a light, fluffy emulsion. Whisk in the coconut oil, then stir in the mashed bananas and vinegar.

Working swiftly now, tip the wet mixture into the dry ingredients and stir as briefly as possible, while ensuring that everything is thoroughly and evenly mixed.

Pour the batter into the prepared loaf pan, and bake in the oven for 10 minutes. Reduce the temperature to 150°C (300°F), and cook for a further 20–25 minutes until the top of the bread is lightly golden and cracked. A skewer or the tip of a sharp knife inserted into the centre of the loaf should come out clean.

Let the banana bread rest in the pan for 5 minutes, before turning out onto a wire rack to cool. Serve slightly warm or cool.

APPLE BUTTER

This simple, versatile preserve can be used as a sauce, a spread, a baby food or even a pie filling. I always make sure that there is apple butter on the breakfast table: it's delicious on toast, with Barley and Oat Groat Porridge (page 56) or Banana Bread (opposite), or alongside Sweet Potato Puffs (page 40). For a special treat, use a spoonful to cap a mountain of soya ice cream. To make this, you'll need a Mouli (rotary food mill) and some preserving (canning) jars. The apple butter will keep, unopened, for a month or two if stored in a cool, dark place.

MAKES 1 LITRE (4 CUPS)

PREPARATION TIME 2 HOURS

12 apples of any type (Bramley, Granny Smith, Cox's Orange Pippin, russet), unpeeled

1 teaspoon ground cinnamon

½ teaspoon grated nutmeg

¼ teaspoon cayenne pepper

50–100g (1¾–2½oz/⅓–⅔ cup, lightly packed) soft light brown sugar, to taste

OPTIONS AND VARIATIONS

You could leave out the cayenne – though this is a rather reluctant suggestion because it's so good for you! Trust me: it brings the flavours together in a pleasing way and doesn't add much heat.

Pour water into a large enamel or stainless-steel saucepan to a depth of 2cm (¾in). Quarter the apples and cut away the tough cores and any bruising or blemishes.

Put the apple quarters in the saucepan. Cover and set over a medium heat until the water starts to simmer. Leaving the pan covered, reduce the heat and allow the apples to cook gently until very tender. This should take about 15 minutes.

Set a Mouli (rotary food mill) over a heatproof bowl. Tip the cooked apples and any juices into the Mouli funnel, and start rotating the handle, one way then the other, until all of the apple flesh has been pushed through the milling plate into the bowl. Scrape the underside of the milling plate to collect all of the purée. Discard the peel and fibrous residue from the Mouli funnel.

Return the puréed apple to the pan and add the spices. Add a little of the sugar, stir well and then sample the purée. Some apples are naturally sweeter than others; you can adjust the amount of sugar that you add until you're happy.

Set the pan over a medium heat and stir well. When the purée starts to bubble and 'puff', reduce the heat to low. Continue cooking, without a lid, to allow the mixture to slowly lose excess moisture. Stir occasionally to prevent sticking or uneven cooking.

When the butter has thickened nicely (after about 1 hour), remove it from the heat. Stir well and ladle the butter into sterilized jars (see below). Seal immediately, and allow to cool.

✳ **PRESERVING (CANNING) JARS** Use wide-mouthed jars with good seals, such as Kilner or mason jars, or any recycled resealable glass jars with tight-fitting lids. Whichever type you choose, make sure that they are sterilized. Wash them thoroughly, including their seals and lids, then fill them with boiling water fresh from a kettle. Leave them standing full of the hot water until you are ready to fill them with your preserve. Empty the water away, fill the jars with the hot butter, and seal them up while still hot.

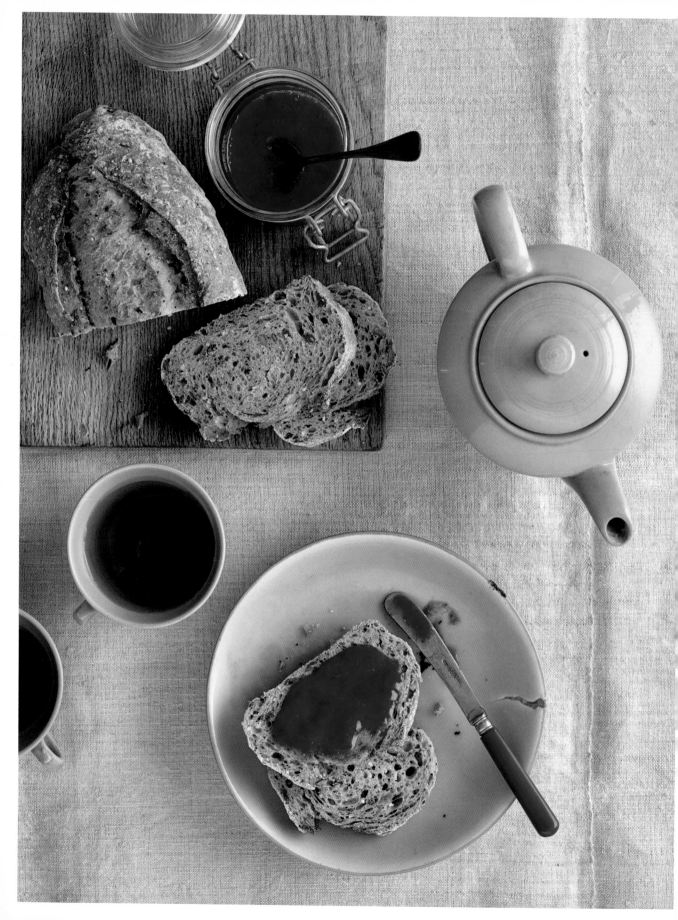

PLUM BUTTER

This variation on Apple Butter (page 43) was the surprise result from a basket of windfall plums. Use whatever type of plum you can find. The flavour and colour of your butter will alter depending on the kind you use – for instance, dark, sweet plums will make a dark, sweet butter. I've been fortunate enough to make this from bullaces – an old variety of plum found in the wild in Britain – and recommend you try them, if you can find them. You'll need a Mouli (rotary food mill) and some preserving (canning) jars. Fruit butters can be used as a sauce, a spread, a topping for desserts, or as a baby food. Try a dollop with Corn and Carrot Muffins (page 35) or Three-Grain Risotto (page 184), or stir a little chilled plum butter into your favourite plain or vanilla soya yogurt.

MAKES ABOUT 1 LITRE (4 CUPS)

PREPARATION TIME 2 HOURS

2kg (4½lb) plums

¼–½ teaspoon Chinese five-spice, to taste

50–100g (1¾–2½oz/⅓–⅔ cup, lightly packed) soft light brown sugar, to taste

OPTIONS AND VARIATIONS

Add 1 unpeeled Bramley or other cooking apple, cored and sliced, during the stewing stage.

Pour water into a large enamel or stainless-steel saucepan to a depth of 2cm (¾in), and set the saucepan over a medium heat. Add the plums, scoring the skin of each with a knife as you do so – this will help them to cook more quickly and evenly.

When the water begins to simmer, cover the pan and reduce the heat. Let the plums cook, stirring occasionally, for 15–20 minutes until softened. Remove the pan from the heat and scoop out and discard the stones (pits), which will have separated from the plums (it's important to remove these before putting the cooked plums through the Mouli).

Set the Mouli over a heatproof bowl, and put the cooked plums into the Mouli's funnel. Rotate the mill, one way then the other, until all the plum flesh is pushed through the milling plate into the bowl. Scrape the underside of the plate to collect all of the purée. Discard the residue of skins left behind in the Mouli funnel.

Return the plum purée to the pan. Add the five-spice powder and sugar to taste, bearing in mind that the reducing process will intensify the plums' natural sweetness.

Stir well and set the pan over a medium heat. Continue cooking, without a lid, to allow the purée to slowly lose excess moisture. Stir occasionally to prevent sticking or uneven cooking.

When the butter has thickened nicely (after about 1 hour), remove the pan from the heat. Stir well and ladle the butter into sterilized jars (see note on page 43). This will keep unopened for a month or two if kept in a cool, dark place. This will keep, unopened, for a month or two if kept in a cool, dark place.

ONION AND POTATO FLIP

As part of a hot breakfast or for that starving-hungry-just-got-home moment, this dish is quick and satisfying. The most demanding part, for me, is the flip. When I was a girl, we had a large, flat iron griddle plate that took up half the stovetop. I loved cooking on it: all that space gave me plenty of room to manoeuvre the spatula – and my elbows – to get the perfect angle for the flip. It's a little trickier with a frying pan or skillet, but the popularity of this recipe means that I get plenty of practice! Use raw or cooked potatoes, or a mixture of both, as suits your situation. Make four individual flips or one or two large ones that you can divide. Delicious served with a portion of Stalybridge Beans-on-Toast (page 52) or Broccoli Almond Sizzle (page 190).

SERVES 4

PREPARATION TIME 20 MINUTES

2 medium potatoes, raw, cooked or partially cooked

1 small onion, quartered and thinly sliced

¼ teaspoon crushed caraway seeds

1 tablespoon untoasted sesame oil

Salt and pepper, to taste

OPTIONS AND VARIATIONS

Add ½ teaspoon dried basil or oregano to the potato mixture.

Grate the potatoes into a bowl. Add the onion and caraway seeds, season with salt and pepper, and mix gently using a wooden spoon.

Drizzle the oil into a frying pan (skillet) set over a medium heat. When the oil is hot, spoon the potato mixture into the centre of the pan and spread it out to cover the bottom. Cook for 5 minutes; do not cover the pan.

Using a wooden spoon, draw the ingredients into a cake with a thickness of 1–2cm (½–¾in); wet the wooden spoon to prevent the ingredients sticking to it. Ensure that the onion slices are nicely embedded in the potato and not dangling loose around the edges.

Continue cooking for about 5 minutes until golden on the bottom. Use a spatula to loosen and flip the cake, leaving it to cook and turn golden on the other side for about 5 minutes. Serve hot.

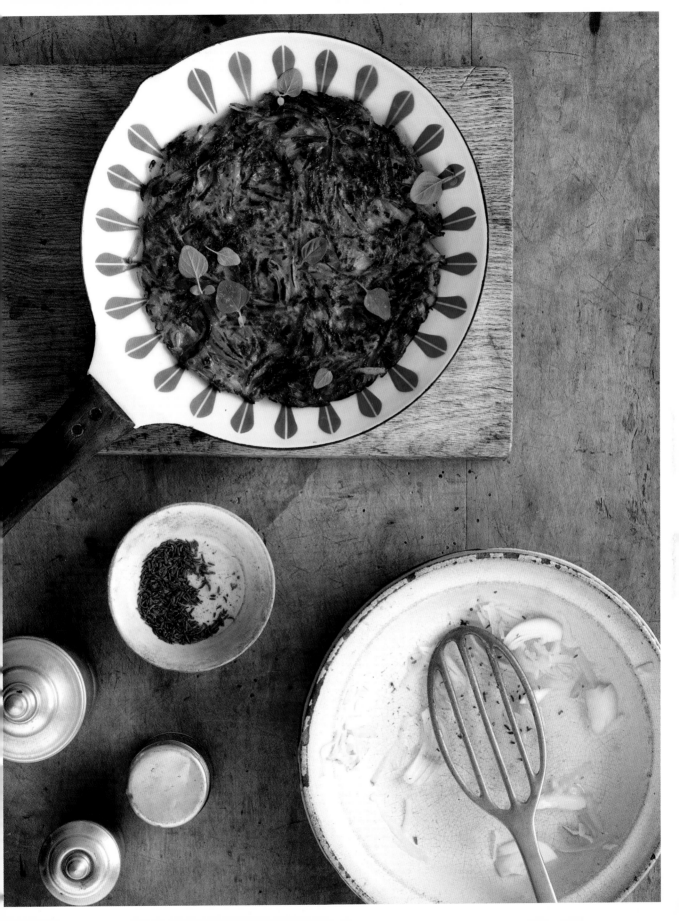

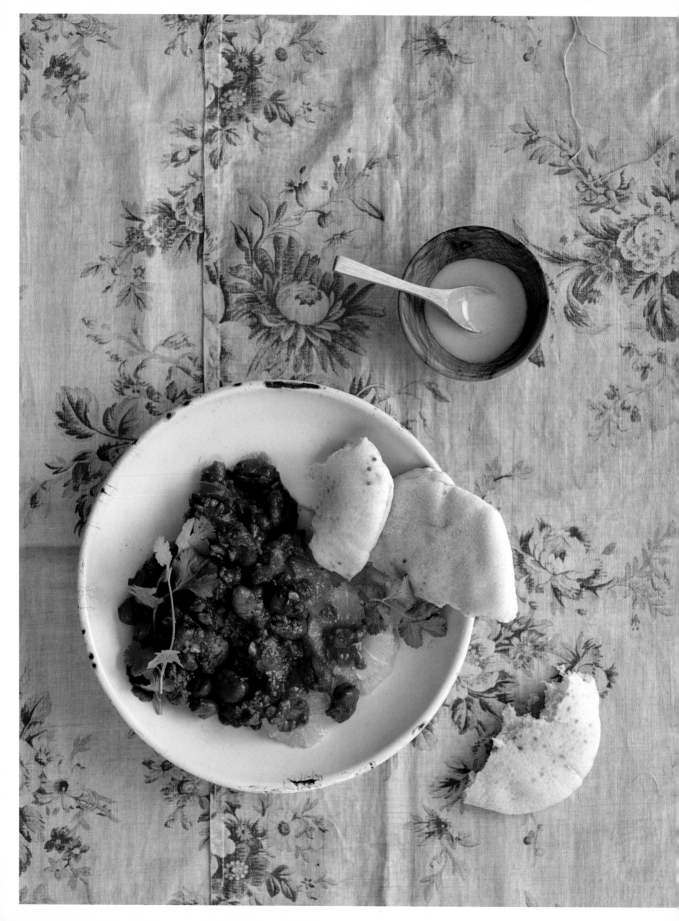

FUL MEDAMES WITH TAHINI AND ORANGE

Ful medames – also known as broad beans or fava beans – have a rugged outer texture and orange-brown colouring. They're among the earliest foods to have been cultivated by humans and an important ingredient in Middle Eastern cuisine – *ful medames* is also the name of a traditional Egyptian breakfast. This dish is fortifying, hot or cold, served with toasted pitta bread or alongside Bubble 'n' Squeak (page 53).

(page 53).

SERVES 4

PREPARATION TIME 30 MINUTES

1 tablespoon untoasted sesame oil

8 garlic cloves, chopped

½ teaspoon cumin seeds

½ teaspoon ground cinnamon

½ teaspoon chilli flakes

1 medium tomato, finely chopped

2 × 400g (14oz) cans ful medames (broad or fava beans)

1 orange, peeled and separated into segments

4 tablespoons tahini

OPTIONS AND VARIATIONS

Add 2 large handfuls of fresh coriander (cilantro) leaves, chopped, when you add the tomato; or 2 finely chopped spring onions (scallions) when you add the beans.

Pour the oil into a large saucepan, and sauté the garlic and spices over a low to medium heat until the garlic is tender, about 5 minutes. Add the chopped tomato and any of its juices, and cook for another 5 minutes, stirring frequently. Add the canned beans and their sauce, stir well, and cook for a further 5 minutes to heat through.

Remove the pan from the heat. Slice the orange segments into bite-sized chunks and stir them into the hot beans. Drizzle a spoonful of tahini over each portion of beans and oranges, and serve.

✳ **RUGGED AND RELIABLE** I've noticed that foods with a long history and somewhat undistinguished appearance are often especially nutritious. Ful medames are just such a food: they are rich in protein, iron, magnesium and manganese, as well as being high in both soluble and insoluble fibre. These wonderful beans have a rugged outer texture and orange-brown colouring when dried. The preparation of dried beans is not always convenient in the breakfast rush – but, fortunately, you can buy cooked ful medames in cans, as used in this recipe.

QUICK PATTY CAKE MIX

This versatile concoction is so handy: just add water and shape into sausages, burgers – or even a celebration roast (see below)! I make a big batch of the dry mix and store it in a glass jar so that it's always ready when I need it. As burgers, they make a tasty meal with Onion and Potato Flip (page 46) and Sweetcorn and Pepper Relish (page 134). As sausages, they look traditional beside a portion of Stalybridge Beans-on-Toast (page 52) for a hearty cooked breakfast.

MAKES 4 BURGERS OR SAUSAGES

PREPARATION TIME 30 MINUTES

2 tablespoons dried onion

2 tablespoons rice flakes

2 tablespoons oat flakes (rolled oats)

2 tablespoons oat bran

2 tablespoons fine couscous

1 tablespoon vegan gravy powder

1 teaspoon dried oregano

½ teaspoon cayenne pepper

2 tablespoons untoasted sesame oil

A little plain (all-purpose) flour, for dusting

OPTIONS AND VARIATIONS

To make a spicier version, double the amount of cayenne or add ½ teaspoon chilli flakes instead. Add interest, bulk and texture to the basic mixture by adding 100g (3½oz/about ½ cup) cooked rice, cooked potatoes, cooked beans or tofu chunks. Get creative and try adding extra spices or herbs, too.

In a bowl, stir together the dried onion flakes, rice flakes, oat flakes, oat bran, couscous, gravy powder, oregano and cayenne pepper. Add 125ml (4fl oz/½ cup) warm water, stir well and leave to stand for 10 minutes.

Sprinkle a little flour onto a chopping board. Divide the soaked mixture into four, and shape into burger or sausage-shaped patties on the floured board. If they are burgers, turn them so that both sides get a light coating of flour. If they are sausages, roll them to coat lightly all over with flour.

Pour half the oil into a frying pan (skillet) set over a medium heat. When hot, add the burgers or sausages, and cover the pan. Cook for 5 minutes until browned and slightly crisp, then turn them and cook the other side (or sides) in the same way, adding more oil if needed. When the patties are nicely browned, reduce the heat and cook for 10 minutes, turning occasionally to prevent them sticking or burning.

VEGAN ROAST Patty Cake Mix can be used to make a tasty oven-baked roast as a centrepiece for a family dinner. To feed 4 people, put double quantities of the dry ingredients from the recipe above into a large bowl. Stir in 250ml (9fl oz/1 cup) warm water and leave to stand for 10 minutes. Add about 250g (9oz) cooked beans, mashing them slightly as you stir them in. Press the mixture into an oiled loaf pan or a fancy baking mould. Cover the upper surface of the roast with 150ml (5fl oz/about ⅔ cup) of spicy tomato sauce, such as Rich Tomato Sauce (page 252). Bake at 180°C (350°F) for 35 minutes. Leave to cool in the pan on a wire rack for 5 minutes, then turn out onto a serving plate. Any leftovers can be sliced and fried as part of a hot breakfast, or used as a sandwich filling.

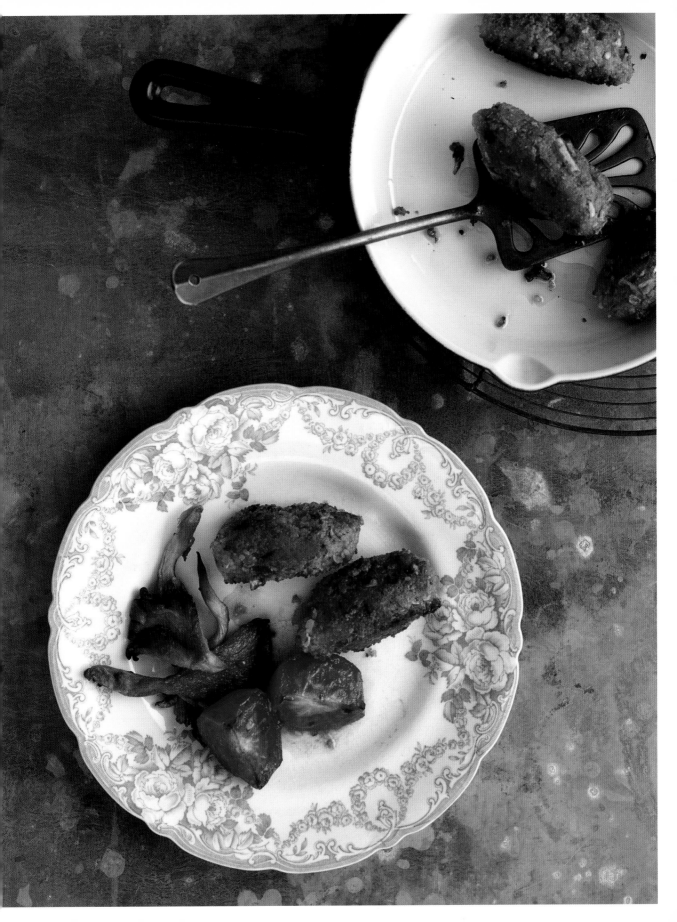

STALYBRIDGE BEANS-ON-TOAST

These beans, cooked outdoors on a camping stove, were our breakfast every morning throughout a fondly remembered family holiday. As we found at the time, every brand of baked beans has a different sauce and flavour, but over that short period the recipe evolved to this, the family-approved standard. It is especially delicious served outdoors or when you have just come in from the cold. At home, we serve the beans on slices of toasted Splendid Wholesome Loaf (page 120).

SERVES 4

PREPARATION TIME 15 MINUTES

1 tablespoon untoasted sesame oil

1 large onion, finely chopped

¼ teaspoon chilli flakes

¼ teaspoon ground allspice

1 medium tomato, finely chopped

2 × 415g (14oz) cans baked beans

4 thick slices of bread, toasted

OPTIONS AND VARIATIONS

Add ¼ teaspoon ground turmeric with the spices. This will change the colour and flavour a little, and thicken the sauce, too.

Pour the oil into a saucepan, and sauté the onion over a medium heat. Add the spices and chopped tomato, cover the pan and leave to cook for about 5 minutes.

When the onion and tomato are tender, add the baked beans and stir well. Cook gently to warm the beans while you toast the bread, then remove from the heat. Ladle the beans over the toast and serve.

✱ **CANNED VERSUS DRIED** I was surprised to learn that canned food has been around since the early nineteenth century, as part of the everlasting quest to find ways of making foods stay viable for longer. The method proved successful, with a few glitches along the way, and was 'big business' by the middle of that century. Currently, canned goods have the second-highest carbon footprint, after frozen foods. That makes sense when you consider the resource materials required, the manufacturing, and the transport involved. In addition, people often store canned food but don't use it before the sell-by-date. Not only is the food wasted, the can is wasted, too, because it is unlikely to be recycled. A sack of dried beans minimizes the carbon footprint of a bean-based meal. I buy dried beans in preference to canned ones for several other reasons, too. I can find more variety, they keep really well, and they are much cheaper. I can get about 12 meals for four out of a 2kg (4½ lb) sack of dried beans and maybe one meal out of a 400g (14oz) can. Cans are handy, especially on a camping trip or for exotic ingredients, and I do use canned foods from time to time. However, fresh foods remain my first choice, with dried foods as the favourite for anything that is likely to require longer periods of storage.

BUBBLE 'N' SQUEAK

Not so much a recipe as a response to leftovers from a roast dinner, this dish is a classic that's never the same twice, but always starts with an onion. Traditionally served as part of a cooked breakfast, it's good at any time of day. You can include just about any vegetable you have to hand in this dish. However, the results should not be oily or charred, but fairly dry with each ingredient distinct. Top with your favourite bottled sauce or a dash of tamari. Serve with a sausage made from Quick Patty Cake Mix (page 50) and perhaps a grilled tomato.

SERVES 4

PREPARATION TIME 20 MINUTES

1 tablespoon untoasted sesame oil

1 large onion, finely chopped

2 baked or roasted potatoes, coarsely chopped

1 roasted parsnip, chopped

1 roasted carrot, chopped

100g (3½oz) fresh Brussels sprouts, trimmed and quartered

100g (3½oz/⅔ cup) fresh or frozen green peas

1 cabbage leaf, finely sliced or chopped

½ teaspoon dried oregano

Salt and pepper, to taste

Pour the oil into a large frying pan (skillet) set over a medium-high heat. Add the onion, potatoes, parsnip, carrot, Brussels sprouts, green peas, cabbage and oregano, layering the vegetables in the order given and seasoning to taste with the salt and pepper as you go. Cover the pan. Do not stir – yet.

Cook for about 5 minutes until the onion is beginning to brown, then use a spatula to turn the contents of the pan so that the onion and potatoes are uppermost. Cover the pan, reduce the heat and cook for a further 5 minutes until the sprouts are tender.

Stir well and serve hot.

SAFETY FIRST It's great to use up leftovers and avoid waste, but crucial to practise food safety.

* Store cooked or perishable foods at temperatures below 5°C/40°F and use them as soon as possible.

* Do not keep cooked foods at room temperature for longer than 2 hours.

* When reheating cooked foods, always bring them to full heat (above 60°C/140°F) before serving.

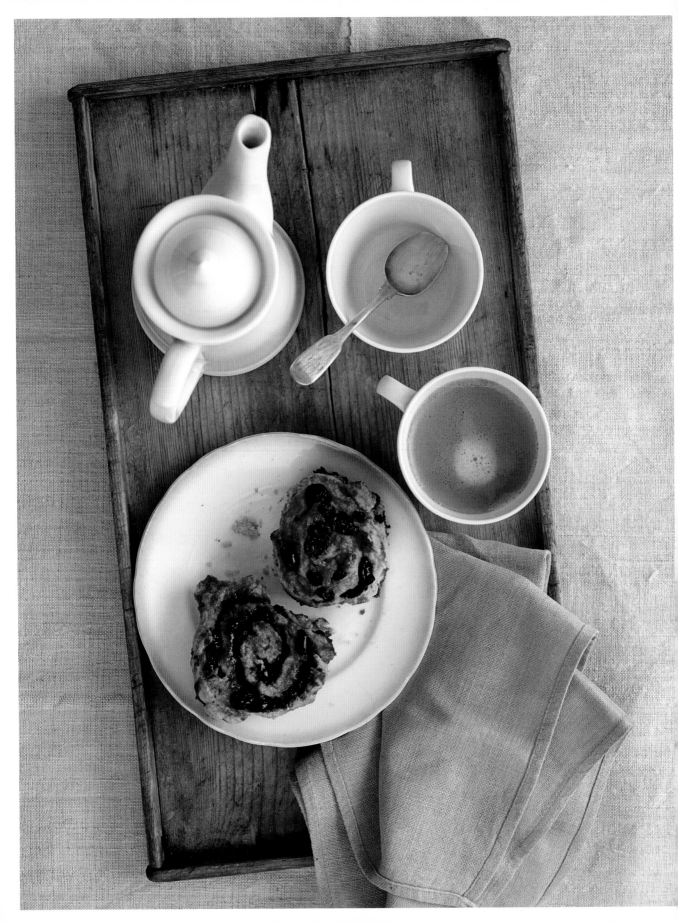

SWEET SUNDAY ROLLS

Although these are quick to prepare, it's a pleasure to take your time making them and to serve them as a bit of a treat. They're perfect for a relaxed Sunday morning with a pot of coffee and the newspapers, and perhaps a bowl of fresh berries.

SERVES 4

PREPARATION TIME 40 MINUTES

40g (1½oz/½ cup) desiccated (shredded) coconut

100g (3½oz/½ cup, lightly packed) soft light brown sugar

1 teaspoon ground cinnamon

300g (10½oz/2½ cups) plain (all-purpose) or wholemeal (whole-wheat) flour, plus extra for dusting your work surface

2 teaspoons bicarbonate of soda (baking soda)

1 teaspoon cream of tartar

80g (2¾oz) coconut oil, plus a little extra for greasing the dish

150ml (5fl oz) plant milk

100g (3½oz/⅔ cup) raisins

2 tablespoons extra virgin olive oil

90ml (3fl oz) maple or barley malt syrup

OPTIONS AND VARIATIONS

Drizzle a little extra virgin olive oil over the rolls before baking them, to create a slightly crispy surface.

Preheat the oven to 220°C (425°F), and grease a 28cm (11¼in) round baking dish or similar ovenproof dish with a generous coating of coconut oil. Sprinkle the desiccated coconut over the greased dish, jostling it a little to distribute evenly.

Combine the sugar and cinnamon in a small bowl. Sprinkle half of the cinnamon sugar over the coconut-coated baking dish.

In a separate bowl, mix the flour, bicarbonate of soda and cream of tartar. Add the coconut oil and use a table knife to 'cut' it into the dry ingredients until the mixture resembles fine breadcrumbs. Add the plant milk and stir well, then knead to a firm dough using your hands.

Lightly flour a work surface. Turn out the dough and shape it into a rough rectangle. Use a rolling pin (or simply press with your hands) to flatten it into a bigger rectangle of about 20 × 30cm (8 × 12in), with a thickness of about 1.5cm (⅝in).

With the long edge closest to you, spread the raisins over the dough, leaving a gap of about 3cm (1¼in) all around the edges. Lightly press the raisins into the dough. Sprinkle the remaining cinnamon sugar over the raisins, and drizzle with the olive oil and half of the syrup.

Roll the dough into a log from the long edge, working away from you. Press firmly as you roll to ensure that the filling is properly embedded. Check that the ends and the long edge are closed – if necessary, dampen those edges and press together to seal.

Using a serrated bread knife, cut the roll into slices about 3cm (1¼in) thick. Lay the slices flat in the prepared baking dish, leaving a little room between each slice. Bake in the oven for 15 minutes.

While the rolls are baking, cut a piece of baking paper large enough to cover the baking dish. When the rolls are cooked, set the dish on a wire rack or trivet. Lay the baking paper over the dish and put a large plate or tray upside-down on top of the paper, with the baking dish centred underneath. Using oven gloves, carefully lift the dish and plate, holding them firmly together as you turn them over.

Leave the baking dish upside down on the plate for 2–3 minutes, then carefully lift off. Collect and spread any coconut mixture left in the dish over the rolls, which are now upside down. Drizzle the remaining syrup over the rolls while they are still hot. Cool for 10–15 minutes, before gently pulling them away from each other. Eat while still warm.

BARLEY AND OAT GROAT PORRIDGE

At first I found it hard to believe that two tablespoons of grains could yield such a sustaining meal! Take a few minutes in the evening to wash and soak the grains, then have this slow-cook breakfast, knowing that you can go to work or school, and won't 'fade' halfway through the morning. This recipe makes a medium-sized serving that will not overwhelm someone who generally avoids breakfast, but with a few extras it becomes more substantial. For a growing teenager, for instance, you might want to double it. For a sweet porridge, serve with maple syrup, All-Seasons Fruit Salad (page 36) or Apple Butter (page 43). If you prefer a savoury porridge, serve with salt, pepper and olive oil.

SERVES 1

PREPARATION TIME 45 MINUTES + 8 HOURS SOAKING

1 tablespoon pot (hulled) barley

1 tablespoon oat groats

125–200ml (4–7fl oz/½–scant 1 cup) plant milk

OPTIONS AND VARIATIONS

For a lighter porridge, or if you don't have enough milk, cook the porridge with water and add milk only for the last few minutes of cooking.

Measure the grains into a saucepan and wash them in cold water. Drain and rinse again, then cover the grains with fresh cold water to a depth of 2cm (¾in). Leave them to soak for at least 8 hours, but ideally all day or overnight.

Drain and rinse the soaked grains. Put them into a pan with 125ml (4fl oz/½ cup) of the plant milk, and bring to a simmer over a medium heat. Cover the pan, reduce the heat and cook for 25 minutes until the grains are completely softened, stirring from time to time.

With the pan still over a low heat, gradually add more milk to the simmering porridge, stirring after each addition, to create the consistency you desire. Continue to add milk if you prefer a creamier porridge (or if you simply need more time before you are ready to sit down to eat). Both grains can absorb a great deal of liquid.

Serve the porridge hot.

✱ **COOKING WHOLE GRAINS** In my experience, all whole grains (and these in particular) cook best in a pan with a tight-fitting lid that doesn't have a steam hole. After bringing the contents to a simmer, I cover the pan and reduce the heat to very low. In this way, maximum moisture is retained and used to rehydrate the grain: I rarely have to add extra liquid. I also don't have the hassle of clearing a clogged steam hole and the cooking time is usually reduced, sometimes greatly reduced. After you've cooked a certain type of grain once or twice, you'll get a sense of how much liquid to add at the beginning and when is the right time to lift the lid to reveal the tender, cooked grains.

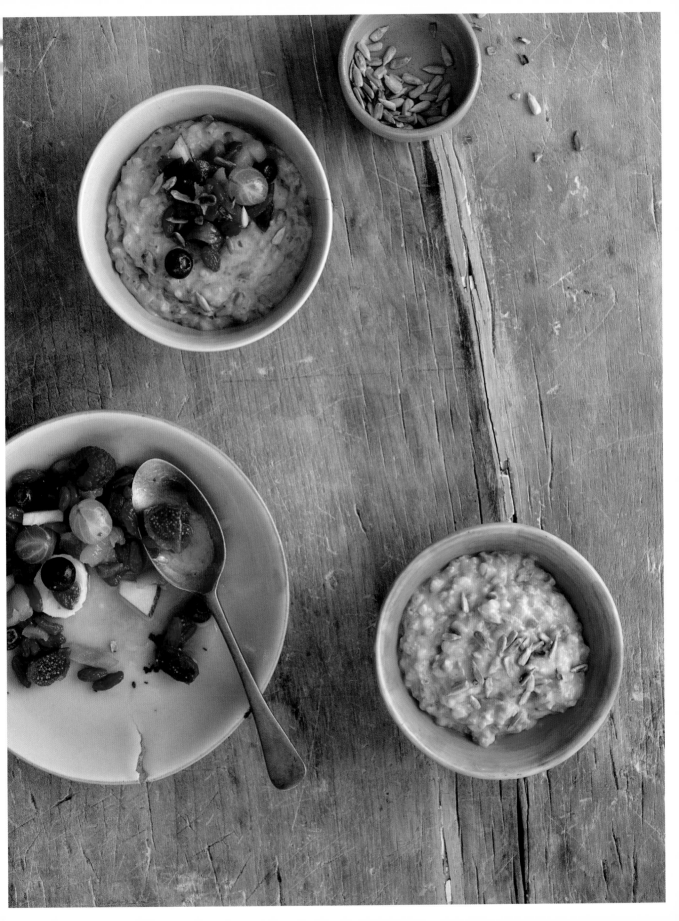

THE VEGAN LARDER

LARDER ESSENTIALS

A useful larder (pantry) is a store of goods that suits you, your family and your kitchen space. It includes all the basics, so that you can make a meal anytime, and a few special items to give you creative scope. Store fresh and perishable goods in the refrigerator and replace them weekly. Store nonperishable foods in a cool, dry place that is also out of direct light. Clean your larder once each season to prevent an accumulation of old foods and rotate your stock — older packets, jars or cans should be pulled forward for more immediate use. Here are foods to stock:

DRIED FRUITS are a handy snack, or can be chopped into a salad or onto cereal. Cook them into a curry or add them to a chutney. They are flavour-intense and mineral-rich.

DRIED HERBS AND SPICES let you create delicious flavour combinations. Buy three or four of each and start experimenting.

DRIED VEGETABLES can be very useful. Dried onion or garlic can be used in marinades and are included in Quick Patty Cake Mix (page 50). Dried mushrooms keep for years and have an exquisite flavour. Dried tomatoes have an intense flavour and are versatile. They keep for months rather than years.

FRESH FRUIT AND VEGETABLES are perishable. Our family visits the farmers' market every Sunday to buy a week's supply. Fruit and greens are thoroughly washed before storing (this saves a load of time on meal prep during the week). Greens, berries and roots are kept in the refrigerator; the rest create colourful arrangements on the work counter or kitchen table.

PLANT MILKS are available from most supermarkets, as well as organic grocers and health food stores. There is soya milk, of course, but also grain milks, from oats or rice; nut milks made from almond, cashew or coconut; and seed milks such as sunflower, hemp or sesame. Each milk has its own flavour and nutrient profile: all are rich in minerals and provide protein, fat and simple carbohydrates. Some brands are fortified with vitamin D or calcium or B_{12}. In our family, we use almond and soya milks most often, followed by oat and hemp. Sometimes we even make our own!

SALT always starts with sea salt, but try tamari, black salt and ume shiso.

SEA VEGETABLES are available in dried form and are rich in minerals. My four essentials are: Agar-agar is a flavourless thickener that can replace gelatine (an animal product) to make jellies. Arame, once briefly soaked and cooked, gives a distinctive but not overpowering flavour to salads, casseroles or sautés. Kombu strips help to soften beans as they cook, deepen the flavour of soups and broths, and enhance their nutrient profile. Nori flakes, sprinkled over any dish, add nutrient value, a delicate flavour and visual appeal; nori sheets are used to wrap sushi or sold as a crispy snack food.

SYRUPS such as barley malt and molasses are a must; carob and pomegranate syrups are treats.

VINEGAR should be apple cider or wine to begin with, then start exploring.

GRAINS AND FLOURS

These are staple foods, rich in nutrients, flavour and appeal. Store them in airtight containers away from the light and use within one year.

RICE grows all over the world, comes in a great many varieties, is easy to store and keeps well. The quickest to cook are basmati and jasmine rice, both of which are 'white' rices, but long- or short-grain whole brown rice is a healthier staple, rich in minerals and fibre, with a nutty flavour. It takes slightly longer to cook than the white rices. Arborio is a white rice used for risotto and rice pudding. It should not be washed and absorbs more liquid than other rices. Rice flakes are grains of rice rolled flat, rather like oat flakes (rolled oats). These flakes are useful in bean butters, breads or sauces, and are an excellent base for introducing semisolid foods to infants. Wild rice is dark brown with a strong, earthy flavour and aroma.

HOW TO COOK WHOLE GRAINS

* 70–100g (2½–3½oz/½–¾ cup) dry grain is sufficient for a serving per person.
* Wash and drain the grain, tip into a saucepan and cover to twice its depth in fresh water; place over a medium heat. When the water begins to simmer, cover the pan, reduce the heat and leave to cook for 25–30 minutes.
* Option: soak grains for 4–12 hours prior to cooking; drain and rinse, cook as above.

OATS are a highly nutritious grain, rich in soluble fibre and very easy to digest. They have many uses, but are most commonly used to make porridge. Oats in groat, rolled (flake) or steel-cut form are all generally considered to be whole.

BARLEY in its whole form is called 'pot' (hulled) barley and is far more nutritious than 'pearl' barley, especially if you soak it (1–4 hours) before cooking. It can be served with a topping of bean or vegetable stew, made into porridge or included in a sustaining winter soup.

BUCKWHEAT has a very earthy flavour and a dense texture. It's not a form of wheat, despite its name, and is naturally gluten-free. In its whole groat form, cook in the same way as rice or barley. It can be mixed with other grains, such as rice or millet, to create a dish with colour and texture variations.

MILLET is a round, white grain. It is nutrient-rich, stores well and contributes a unique texture and creamy-white appearance to any meal. It can take longer to cook than you might suppose – usually the same length of time as wholegrain (brown) rice.

CORN (maize) is sold in fine, medium or coarse 'grinds' or 'meals', and is used to make polenta and cornbread. Cornflour (cornstarch) is made from only the starch of the corn kernel. It is used to thicken sauces and gravies, and also to add sheen to foods cooked in it.

WHEAT is one of the top three most consumed grains in the world (along with rice and maize). It is nutritious but vulnerable to losing much of its nutrient value during refinement, which is done to excess in many cultures. Spelt, kamut and einkorn are ancient varieties of wheat. Spelt is the most readily available of these, as whole grain, flour or pasta. Emmer, also called farro, is another ancient wheat with a nutrient-rich profile. Farro can be harder to find, but try it (usually cooked like rice) if you get the chance. Couscous is a butter-coloured wheat product used in North African cuisine. It is quick to prepare, with a light and pleasing texture that is background to classic stews and sauces. Freekeh is a Middle Eastern and North African wheat product used sparingly in soups and stews. It is green wheat berries that have been sun-dried, roasted and their husks rubbed off.

RYE is a very hardy grain with a long history of use in northern European climates especially. It is dark with a strong, slightly bitter flavour, but is nutrient-rich and sustaining. Experiment with this grain and its flour if you enjoy bread-making.

QUINOA is a recently popularized seed from the Andes in South America. It is especially rich in protein and calcium, and abundant with other vitamins and minerals. Prepare it as you would millet or rice; it is excellent in grain mixtures.

AMARANTH, like quinoa, is exceptionally rich in protein and calcium, and nutrient-dense in general. It has an intense quality, as do many other hardy grains. Cook by itself or blend into breads or grain mixtures. There is a trend to pop it, like popcorn.

TEFF is a minuscule grain grown in Ethiopia and Eritrea in eastern Africa, as well as parts of North America and Australia. It is another powerhouse of nutrients used in grain mixtures, as a cooked breakfast cereal or ground into a flour for breads and cakes. You might need to buy it online.

WHEAT FLOURS include wholemeal (whole-wheat), strong white bread flour, white, self-raising (self-rising), gluten-free, spelt … and so on. If you do any baking or make any basic white sauce, you will need to store one or two of these flours.

RYE FLOUR can be used on its own or blended with other flours to create strong, dark breads.

NATURALLY GLUTEN-FREE FLOURS include quinoa, coconut, rice, corn, oat, gram, millet, potato and buckwheat. Buckwheat flour can make up 25–50 per cent of the flour for breads or batters. Amaranth, quinoa and teff are available as flours; you might need to purchase online. Gram flour is not ground from a grain, but from the chickpea (garbanzo bean). It is commonly used in Indian and some Middle Eastern dishes. Add it to bread flours or pancake batter.

PASTA is generally made from durum wheat, though there are many alternatives, such as spelt, corn and millet. It comes in various shapes and is essentially a dried paste of water and flour.

NOODLES are made in a similar way to pasta, from wheat (ramen and udon), buckwheat (soba), rice (glass or cellophane) or bean flours.

BEANS AND LENTILS

'Beans, beans, the musical fruit,
  The more you eat, the more you toot,
  The more you toot, the better you feel,
  So eat some beans with every meal.'

Let's get the farting sorted out, straight away! It is caused by the natural fermentation of sugars in your large intestine. Like any fermentation, a bit of gas is produced. This is all very natural and beans are not the only cause; cabbage, rye and potatoes are also potential members of the 'orchestra'. In fact, fermentation can be fed by dietary fibre from any source and is variable depending on what you eat and the bacteria living in your intestines. The good news is that useful nutrients are produced by this process and the health of your gut is benefited by an increase in those helpful bacteria (often called probiotics). To reduce flatulence:

* Soak and cook dried beans and lentils as described on page 64.
* Cook beans with a strip of kombu seaweed added to the pot or saucepan. This will soften the beans and reduce the quantity of gas produced.
* Sprout the beans and eat them in salad, sandwich or stir-fry.
* Eat beans in fermented forms such as tempeh, miso, natto or tofu.
* Be patient! After a week or two of eating a daily portion of beans, your body will adjust.

Beans are a fantastic food! Now you can get on with enjoying all the best about them, including the following:

* high in protein, fibre, magnesium, iron, folate and other B vitamins
* low in fat, sodium and calories
* free of cholesterol and gluten
* low glycaemic index (GI) rating, providing slow conversion to blood sugar
* four ½–1 cup servings per week promotes regular, healthy bowel movements

Beans are members of the group of plants called legumes, which produce up to twelve 'grains' or seeds inside a pod. Green peas, green beans and broad (fava) beans are good examples. These are harvested and eaten while they are in their green, or tender, stage.

Pulses are legumes that are harvested after they have dried inside their pods. This category includes lentils and all those other beans, such as haricot (navy), kidney and chickpeas (garbanzo beans), that you can buy in their hard dried form. There are hundreds of varieties of pulses grown around the world.

Growing pulses helps to reduce waste. Worldwide, approximately one-third of food produced for humans is wasted or lost. This occurs for various reasons at harvest, during production and in the consumer phase. Pulses are easy to grow and harvest; they can be stored for a long time, so there is very little waste. This fact increases 'food security' by ensuring that adequate supplies of safe, high-nutrient foods can be produced in nearly every region of the globe and supplied consistently to minimize hunger.

Legumes are of great benefit to the environment.

✳ Nodules on their root system fix nitrogen into the soil, thus improving soil health.

✳ They use less water than many other crops and, because they are deep-rooting, they can share water. This is one way in which they help to promote crop diversity.

✳ They are hardy, versatile and resilient. Some can withstand drought; others deep cold.

✳ They are good for 'marginal' environments with poor soil and inhospitable conditions.

✳ They are water-efficient: for example, to produce 450g (1lb) of pulses requires 43 gallons water whereas 450g (1lb) of beef requires 800-1800 gallons water.

✳ Pulses leave a tiny footprint: 450g (1lb) of lamb produces thirty times more GHGs (greenhouse gases) than 450g (1lb) of lentils.

Pulses are inexpensive, easy to store, look interesting and taste delicious. A 2kg (4½lb) packet can provide up to a dozen family meals. Stocking a variety allows you to select for cooking time, colour and texture.

ESSENTIAL PULSES

RED OR YELLOW 'SPLIT' LENTILS are very quick to cook and do not need much (or any) soaking. They do need a very good rinse, but then will quickly cook into a soup or dhal.

BROWN LENTILS are sometimes called continental or European lentils. They benefit from a 30-minute soak, but then cook quickly, are easy to digest and take on the flavour of any spices you wish to add. Delicious hot or cold, plain or spiced, over grain or added to a salad.

YELLOW OR GREEN 'SPLIT' PEAS are hard legumes that are purchased already split in half. Soak for at least 2 hours but better for 8–12 hours. They make a thick soup or dhal.

ADZUKI BEANS, BLACK TURTLE BEANS, RED BEANS, BLACK-EYED BEANS (PEAS) AND HARICOT (NAVY) BEANS all require 8–12 hours soaking followed by 45–60 minutes cooking in a large pan. Appealing for their colours – red, black, polka-dotted or white – each has a unique texture and flavour.

KIDNEY BEANS AND CHICKPEAS (GARBANZO BEANS) need 8–12 hours soaking, then 30 minutes in a pressure cooker. Add them to cooked dishes or salads. Hummus is made from chickpeas.

DRIED FAVA BEANS (also called broad beans or ful medames) require soaking and then cooking in a pressure cooker. They are a staple in the Middle East, cooked with herbs, garlic, spices and lemon. Eaten young and fresh (not dried), they are pale green and very quick to cook.

MUNG BEANS must be soaked 8–12 hours but then you have a choice: either sprout them or cook them into a spicy dhal or delicious Mung Bean Pâté (page 77).

SOYA BEANS are small, round and very hard, and require soaking and pressure cooking. They have been a staple in China and Southeast Asia for centuries. They contain no starch but are rich in protein, fats and minerals. While they are a nutrient powerhouse, they can be quite bland. So, the first rule of cooking with soya is to add plenty of other flavours. These classic soya products can be used in cooking in a variety of ways. Most of them can be stored, sometimes for years, as with miso and soy sauce.

* Young, green soya beans still in their pods are all the rage as edamame. Serve hot or cold, in their pods, with a little salt and a plate to catch the empty pods.
* Make soya milk from cooked soya beans. Serve sweetened or plain; hot or cold.
* Turn soya milk into tofu, a curd pressed into a soft, silken or firm block. It is versatile, quick to cook and takes on the colour and flavour you give it.
* Soya beans can be fermented into soy sauce. When fermented with wheat, soy sauce is called shoyu; without wheat it is tamari, which is gluten-free.
* Miso paste is made from fermented soya beans, sometimes mixed with rice or barley. It is salty, very nutritious and commonly used to make miso soup, or included in spreads. Buy miso unpasteurized and keep it in a glass jar rather than in plastic, if you can.
* Tempeh (pronounced *tem-pay*) is also made from fermented soya beans. It comes chilled and vacuum-sealed, or in blocks that are deep frozen. Buy it from organic, health foods or speciality grocers for Southeast Asian cuisines. You need to cook tempeh, usually by light frying. It will readily absorb flavours. In fact, it absorbs them so well, adding more spices, herbs or marinade than you expect will be necessary.

HOW TO COOK BEANS

* Pour dried beans into a large saucepan. Wash and drain them, then cover (to twice their depth) with cold water. They will roughly double in size.
* Put the beans aside to soak for 4–12 hours depending on the variety (see page 63 for the different timings).
* Once soaked, pour the beans into a colander, rinse them under cold water and tip them into a pressure cooker or large saucepan. Cover with fresh water.
* Cook the beans in a pressure cooker for 25–30 minutes, or 45–50 minutes in a large pan. Chickpeas (garbanzo beans) require an extra 5 minutes in the pressure cooker.
* Drain and rinse the beans, and add them to your meal.

HOW TO COOK LENTILS

* Wash and drain lentils until the water runs clear.
* Soak for 30 minutes in cold water or for 10 minutes in boiling water.
* Drain and rinse; tip into a saucepan and cover with fresh water.
* Cook for 20–25 minutes. Do not use a pressure cooker as lentils clog the valve!

Beans and lentils love flavour – experiment with the spices and herbs in your larder.

FATS, OILS AND BUTTERS

It's easy to feel bewildered when trying to select healthy fats. Aim for stable fats that don't become rancid quickly, and spend a little extra to ensure they are highest quality.

SESAME OIL is very stable and excellent for most cooking needs. Very little is required and it may be used at high temperatures. Buy sesame oil cold-pressed and unrefined from an ethnic or health food grocer; this oil is not the same as toasted sesame oil.

COCONUT OIL is flavoursome, aromatic and – although free of cholesterol – saturated, and so it is best used in small amounts infrequently. It may be used at high temperatures and keeps well.

OLIVE OIL is not for high-temperature cooking. It is excellent in salad dressings or as an alternative to butter or margarine. Buy extra virgin, organic, cold-pressed, unrefined.

FLAX (FLAXSEED OR LINSEED) OIL is deliciously nutty and aromatic. It is so good for you it should be called medicine. It is not for cooking and, in fact, should be stored in the refrigerator. Drizzle 1–2 tablespoons per day over salads, into smoothies or onto grain dishes. Buy this oil organic, unrefined and cold-pressed, and use within 3 months.

HEMP OIL is second to flax oil but not by much! Use it and store it in the same way.

NUT AND SEED BUTTERS can be used in cooking, as spreads or in dressings. Tahini is made from sesame seeds. Use as a spread or dip, drizzle over hot beans or add spices and serve in a falafel wrap. It emulsifies added liquids. Dark sesame butter or a dark tahini is most nutritious. Peanut butter is nutrient-rich and widely available. As it can trigger an allergic response in some people, you might be wise to withhold this food from very young children. This butter emulsifies added liquids and is an ingredient in sauces from many world cuisines. Favoured are brands that are organic, unsweetened and without added palm oil.

VEGAN MARGARINES are widely available. They are useful on occasion, but are easily replaced by one of the above oils or butters. Select cautiously to avoid consumption of trans fats (trans-fatty acids), also called partially hydrogenated oils. This process turns liquid oils into solid or semisolid fats. After decades of use in margarines, shortenings, baked goods and some snack foods, they have been recognized as being of no value to human health and with no safe level of consumption. The World Health Organization has the goal of eliminating industrially produced trans fats by 2023.

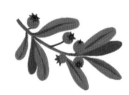

BREAKS AND SNACKS

DIVINE POPCORN

Treat yourself to this wholegrain snack whenever the mood strikes you. It's low-fat, high-fibre, non-GMO – and actually contains useful nutrients. Instead of cooking the corn in a saucepan, you can use an air popper and eliminate the need for any oil. The simple dressing gives the popcorn a delicious, savoury boost and will help any optional extras to coat the kernels nicely. Serve a big bowlful as a snack, or float a handful of popped kernels on the surface of a bowl of soup. They are delicious – a little like croûtons, but much more fun because of the crackling sound they make when they come into contact with the soup.

MAKES 2 LITRES (8 CUPS)

PREPARATION TIME 15 MINUTES

2 tablespoons tamari

1 tablespoon extra virgin olive oil

1 teaspoon apple cider vinegar

¼ teaspoon cayenne pepper

2 tablespoons untoasted sesame oil

100g (3½oz/½ cup) popping corn

OPTIONS AND VARIATIONS

Add a few shakes of hot sauce or Tabasco sauce to the dressing, instead of the cayenne. For extra spiciness, drop 4 whole peppercorns into the dressing. It will gradually take on the spiciness of the pepper. After dressing the popped corn, sprinkle with 2 tablespoons nutritional yeast flakes or 2 tablespoons toasted nori flakes.

Measure the tamari, oil, vinegar and cayenne together into a spray dispenser or shaker bottle.

Heat the sesame oil in a large saucepan over a medium heat. Add the popping corn, cover the pan and let it start to pop. Shake the pan as the corn pops, keeping it on the heat at the same time, until the popping stops after about 5 minutes.

Turn the popped corn into a large bowl. Shake the dressing container, and lightly spray or sprinkle the dressing over the hot corn. Use a wooden spoon to stir the corn, then add a bit more dressing, shaking the dispenser before each use. Serve warm or cold.

* **NORI FLAKES** are little pieces of dried nori, the same seaweed that is used to wrap sushi. Sold in sheets and flakes, and in little strips as a snack food, nori has a broad nutrient profile. It includes useful amounts of iodine when it is consumed on a regular basis. Adding nori to popcorn always gives me a good excuse to make another batch!

* **NUTRITIONAL YEAST FLAKES** are, as their name implies, dried flakes of yeast. Grown on molasses from beet and sugar cane, the yeast is then deactivated so as not to cause digestive problems, but remains a powerhouse of B vitamins, protein, zinc and iron. Some brands are fortified with additional nutrients such as B_{12}. Yeast flakes taste a little like cheese and a little like nuts, adding richness of flavour whether hidden discreetly in a dish or, as in this popcorn, sprinkled in plain sight. Use them in sauces, smoothies and soups.

FRESH OATIES

Oats are a great food that immediately satisfy hunger and can sustain you for a long time. So, when you feel like you have run out of fuel, have one of these bars. Enjoy them with Iced Midsummer Tisane (page 82) or Avocado Almond Shake (see below). One oatie and a small bowl of All-Seasons Fruit Salad (page 36) is almost a meal. They are very simple to make – the perfect project for young cooks.

MAKES 8 SLICES

PREPARATION TIME 45 MINUTES

100g (3½oz) coconut oil, plus extra for greasing the baking tray

75g (2½oz/⅓ cup, firmly packed) soft light brown sugar

2 tablespoons barley malt syrup

½ teaspoon ground cinnamon

200g (7oz/2 cups) oat flakes (rolled oats)

OPTIONS AND VARIATIONS

Add 50g (1¾oz) raisins, sultanas (golden raisins) or mixed candied peel to the pan as you heat the oil and sugar.

Preheat the oven to 150°C (300°F), and lightly oil a 20 × 30cm (8 × 12in) baking tray (sheet pan).

Heat the oil and sugar together in a saucepan and stir until blended. Add the syrup and cinnamon, and stir well. Add the oats, remove from the heat and mix together thoroughly.

Spread the mixture in the prepared baking tray, and bake in the oven for 30 minutes until golden brown. Cut into squares or rectangles while still warm, but leave to cool before serving.

AVOCADO ALMOND SHAKE Beautifully green with a hint of sweetness, this nutritious drink is perfect as an accompaniment to some Fresh Oaties, whether between meals, after a workout or instead of an evening meal. Scoop the flesh of 1 large, ripe avocado into a blender or mixing jug. Add 1 litre (35fl oz/4 cups) chilled almond milk, 2 tablespoons barley malt syrup and 4 teaspoons ground almonds, and blend until smooth. Pour into chilled glasses, sprinkle with a few flaked almonds and serve with a straw and a spoon. If you like, add a tiny pinch of cayenne pepper to the mix, or sprinkle it on top of each portion and give it a swirl with a straw.

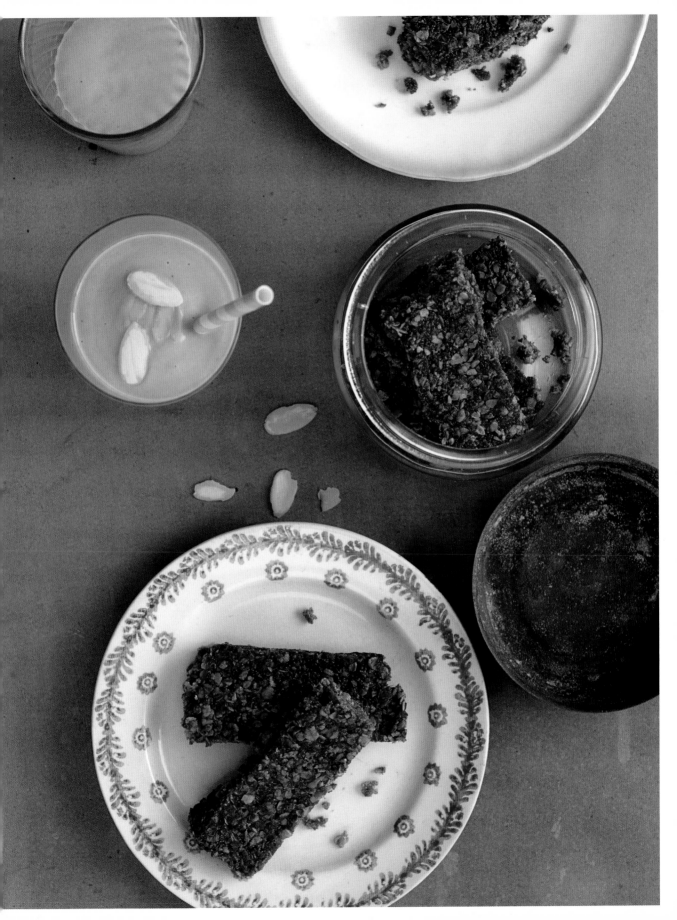

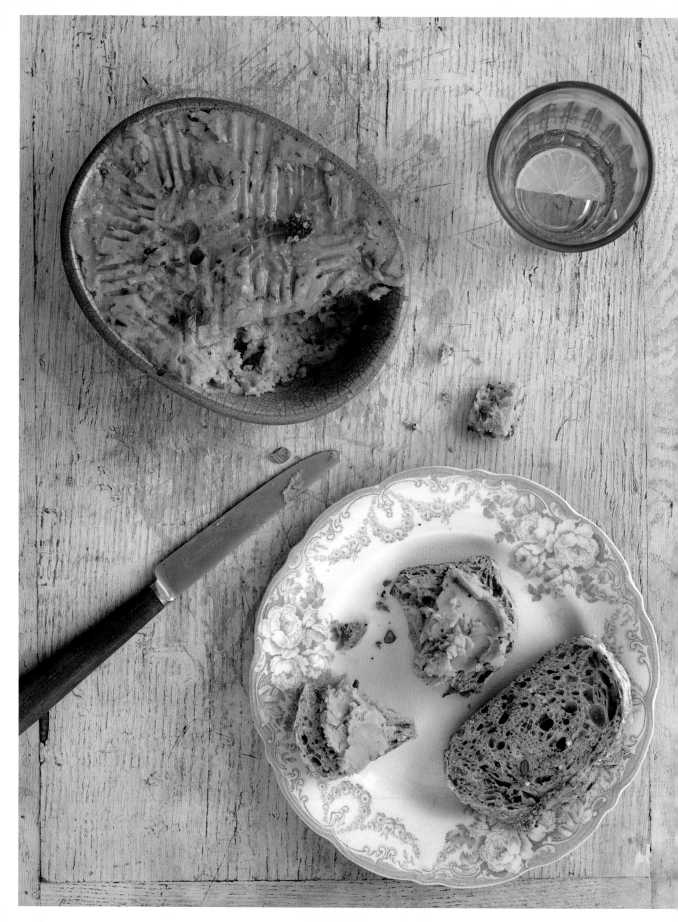

HERB AND ONION BEAN BUTTER

Make this nutritious spread to use in sandwiches or on toast. Double or triple this recipe if you know it will be consumed within the week. It's easy to make and best served chilled. I like to keep mine in an antique butter dish, complete with lid. Serve spread on slices of fresh Seeded Spelt Bread (page 87) or toasted Splendid Wholesome Loaf (page 120).

MAKES ABOUT 250ml (1 CUP)

PREPARATION TIME 40 MINUTES

1 tablespoon untoasted sesame oil

1 medium onion, finely chopped

250g (9oz) cooked white beans such as haricot (navy), cannellini or butter (lima) beans

½ teaspoon dried herbs of your choice (see below)

¼ teaspoon ground turmeric

Pinch of salt

1 tablespoon nutritional yeast flakes

Extra virgin olive oil for drizzling

OPTIONS AND VARIATIONS

Try strong herbs such as thyme or sage, or mild herbs such as parsley or basil. If you prefer, just before leaving the pan to stand for 10 minutes, add 1 tablespoon chopped fresh herbs such as fennel fronds or chives.

Pour the oil into a small saucepan with 1 tablespoon water. Add the onion, cover the pan and cook over a low heat for 10 minutes.

Add the white beans and your choice of herbs, directly on top of the onions, without stirring. Your aim is to cook the onions without browning them, while just warming and softening the beans. Cover the pan and continue cooking over a low heat for a further 10 minutes.

Add the turmeric and pinch of salt, and stir well. Cover the pan and remove from the heat. Leave to stand for 10 minutes, then mash the mixture, adding the yeast flakes as you do so.

Turn the mixture into a covered butter dish or bowl, and press the mixture firmly and evenly into the dish. Leave to cool.

Drizzle a little olive oil over the surface of the bean butter. With a table knife, score the surface back and forth. Serve chilled.

Between servings, keep the dish, covered, in the refrigerator.

AVOCADO PRESS

Make this spread in early summer when the avocados are in season. It will keep, covered, in the refrigerator for two days – though in my experience it usually disappears in one! Serve it with Eat-It-Today Cornbread (page 135) or toasted slices of Splendid Wholesome Loaf (page 120), or use it to augment a Kohlrabi and Cucumber Sandwich (page 123).

MAKES 200ml (7fl oz)

PREPARATION TIME 15 MINUTES

+ 30 MINUTES CHILLING

2 medium, ripe avocados

Juice of 1 lemon

¼ teaspoon cayenne pepper

3 tablespoons finely chopped fresh coriander (cilantro) leaves

1 medium tomato

Salt, to taste

OPTIONS AND VARIATIONS

Sprinkle the top with herb salt or celery salt, instead of ordinary salt.

Scoop the flesh of the avocados into a bowl, removing any blackened or stringy parts. Roughly mash the avocado using a fork, stirring in the lemon juice, cayenne and half of the coriander. Press the mixture into a serving dish, preferably one with a lid.

Finely chop the tomato. Scrape it, and all its juices, on top of the avocado mixture and spread it out evenly. Scatter the remaining coriander over the tomato, and sprinkle with salt.

Cover the dish and refrigerate until ready to use. If you can, give the spread at least 30 minutes to chill, so that the flavours can mature.

GREAT GUACAMOLE

Start here and gradually devise your own version of a fantastic traditional dish. Look for those really big avocados with smooth skin, and tuck them under the bananas in your fruit basket. Rotate them each day and they will ripen beautifully. Divide the batch of guacamole among small bowls and serve with a Crudités Platter (page 239) and warm pitta bread, or Eat-It-Today Cornbread (page 135).

SERVES 4

PREPARATION TIME 20 MINUTES

300g (10oz/1¼ cups) plain, unsweetened soya yogurt

2 garlic cloves, crushed

¼ teaspoon chilli flakes

2 large, ripe avocados

Salt, to taste

OPTIONS AND VARIATIONS

Add a thinly sliced fresh chilli. It is pretty, though very spicy. Or add a couple of finely chopped coriander (cilantro) leaves for a fresh 'note' in the flavours. Adjust the amount of garlic and chilli to suit your taste.

Blend together the yogurt, garlic and chilli flakes in a bowl.

Cut the avocados in half along their length, lift out the stones (pits) and set them aside (see note below). Scoop the flesh into the bowl with the yogurt mixture, discarding any dark or stringy parts.

Use a fork or hand-held blender to work the avocado and yogurt mixture together. The fork will deliver a chunkier texture; the blender a very smooth one.

Just before serving (and not before), stir in the salt. If there is any guacamole left after the meal has ended (very rarely), put the reserved avocado stones into the bowl with it, cover the dish and refrigerate. The stones will help the guacamole to keep its green colour.

GARDEN NETTLE SOUP

Young nettle shoots, available from many local or farmers' markets, give this soup an intense, deep-green colour. Wear gloves or use kitchen tongs when preparing the uncooked nettles, but don't worry – the sting disappears with cooking. Nettles improve the soil, support wildlife and are beneficial to humans, too. Historically, they were one of the wild greens that provided tonic nutrients in early spring, just when they were most needed. Serve with a chunk of Splendid Wholesome Loaf (page 120), ready to wipe the bowl clean.

SERVES 4

PREPARATION TIME 1 HOUR

About 50g (1¾oz) fresh, young nettle shoots (untrimmed weight)

1 tablespoon untoasted sesame oil

1 medium potato, diced

1 leek, chopped

1 onion, chopped

1 celery stalk, chopped

1 teaspoon vegan bouillon powder

¼ teaspoon black pepper

¼ teaspoon ground cinnamon

1 litre (35fl oz/4 cups) vegetable stock or water

Soak the nettles in a sink full of very cold water while you prepare the other ingredients.

Measure the oil into a large stockpot or saucepan set over a medium heat. Add the potato, spreading it out to make a layer in the pan, then make layers of leek, onion and celery. Sprinkle over the bouillon powder, pepper and cinnamon, and cover the pan. Leave to cook for about 20 minutes, stirring once or twice during that time, until the vegetables are tender.

Meanwhile, use kitchen scissors to cut the nettle leaves from their thick stalks; discard the stalks.

When the vegetables in the pan are tender, add the nettle leaves. Cover the pan and cook for about 5 minutes to let the nettles soften and reduce, then stir the leaves into the other vegetables.

Add the stock and purée the soup to your preferred texture using a blender. Bring to a simmer.

Serve immediately, or leave the soup to cool and refrigerate for the next day. Reheat before serving.

✱ **NETTLES** are best eaten in the spring, when they are tender and fresh, and must not be eaten once they have flowered. To collect nettles, wear gloves and carry scissors and a bowl or bag. Cut here and there in a swathe of plants, taking just the growing tips of non-flowering stems. Do not pull the plant from the ground and don't cut so much from one plant that it might have trouble recovering. Avoid plants that might have been sprayed (such as those growing near crops) or those that are close to a road. Soak your picked nettles in cold water before use, and, when you are ready to cook them, lift them stem by stem from the water. This will ensure that any debris is left behind in the soaking water, which should then be discarded.

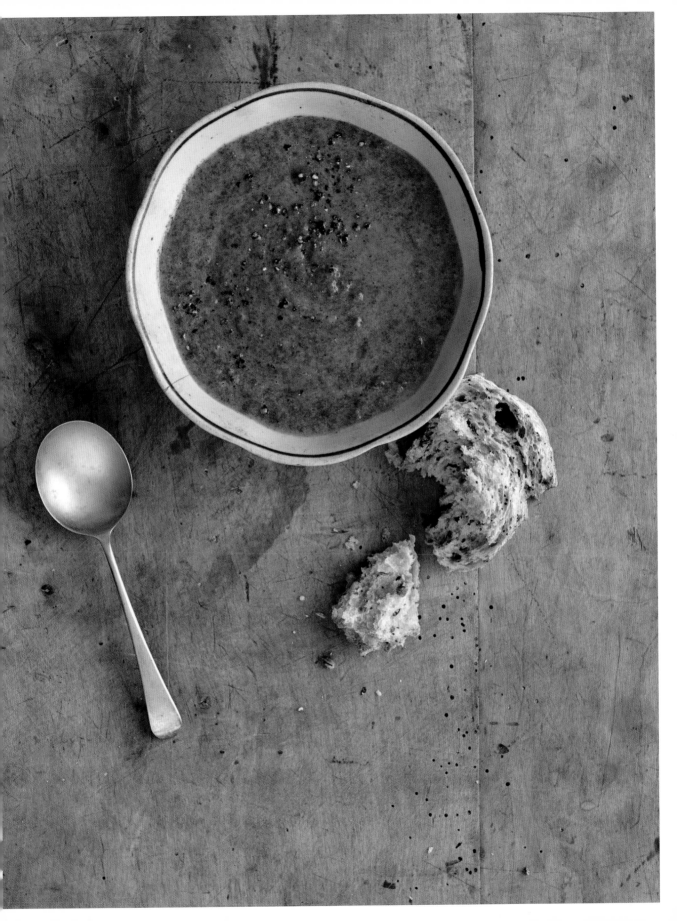

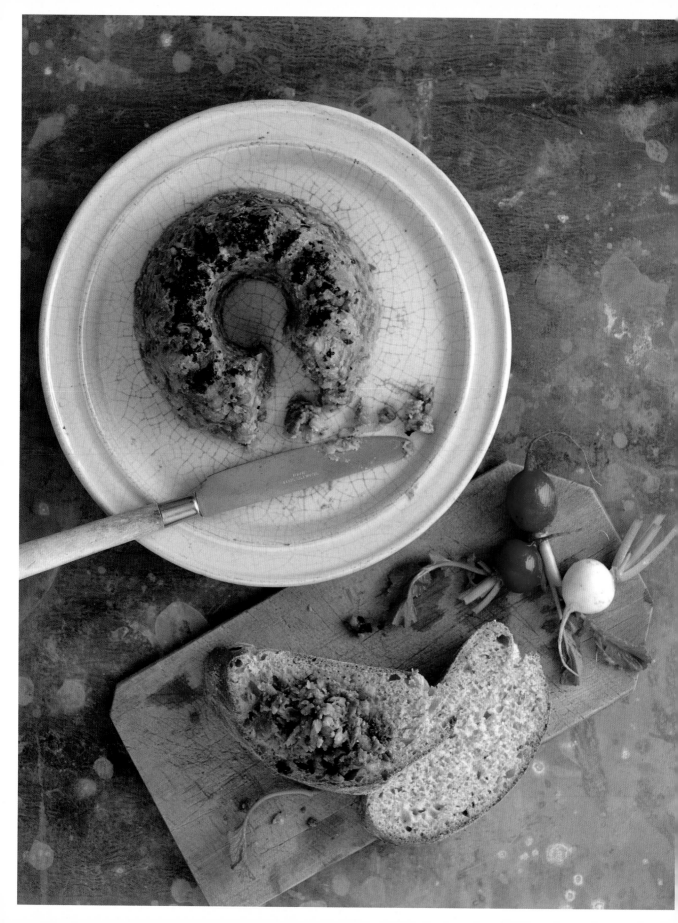

MUNG BEAN PÂTÉ

Serve this delicious bean pâté spread on crackers or toast, or add a thick slice to a hearty cooked breakfast. Mung beans absorb spices, sometimes so much that it is hard to taste them. The quantities of spices listed here will ensure that their flavours are not lost, but feel free to adjust to suit your taste. Use a decorative mould if you have one, to make the pâté into a centrepiece for a buffet lunch or picnic. Serve with Quickly Salad (page 93) and fresh bread such as Rosemary Twist (page 164).

Drain and rinse the soaked mung beans. Put them in a saucepan, and cover with water to a depth of 3cm (1¼in) above their surface. Cover the pan and bring to a low simmer over a medium heat.

Cook for 20 minutes, then check that there is still sufficient water by gently stirring the beans. Their skins should be split, but they will not be fully tender. Add more water as needed, so that it is visible just below the surface of the beans. Cover the pan and cook for a further 10–15 minutes. The beans should be tender and hold their shape until you begin to stir them, then they will break down into a creamy texture. Cover the pan and remove from the heat.

Pour the 2 tablespoons oil into another saucepan set over a medium heat. Add the onion and sauté for about 10 minutes until tender. Add the spices and bouillon powder. Stir well, cover the pan and remove from the heat.

Grind the flaxseeds using a mortar and pestle, or a spice grinder. Mix the ground seeds with the oat bran and yeast flakes. Add this mixture to the sautéed onion and stir well.

Tip the pan to drain the cooked beans of any standing water, if necessary, then add them to the sautéed mixture. Stir well to combine. The beans will lose their shape as you stir them and the dry ingredients will begin to absorb moisture.

Lightly oil a pudding basin or decorative mould, and dust the oiled surface with the nori flakes. Press the bean mixture into the basin or mould, and chill for at least 4 hours, if possible.

To serve, cover the dish with a serving plate and, holding the plate in place, turn over the dish and plate. If the pâté does not drop onto the plate immediately, leave to stand – it should release after 1–2 minutes.

MAKES ABOUT 750ml (3 CUPS)

PREPARATION TIME 1 HOUR +

SOAKING AND CHILLING

250g (9oz/1¼ cups) dried mung beans, soaked (see How to Cook Beans, page 64)

2 tablespoons untoasted sesame oil, plus extra for oiling the basin or mould

1 medium onion, finely chopped

1 teaspoon Chinese five-spice

1 teaspoon ground ginger

1 teaspoon black pepper

1 teaspoon vegan bouillon powder

2 tablespoons flaxseeds (linseeds)

2 tablespoons oat bran

2 tablespoons nutritional yeast flakes

2 tablespoons nori flakes

OPTIONS AND VARIATIONS

Try dusting the mould with 2 tablespoons sumac instead of the nori flakes. For a pleasing presentation, divide the pâté into two portions and press into two separate small moulds, one dusted with nori flakes (dark green), the other with sumac (deep red).

SPROUTED MUNG BEANS

You can make fresh sprouts all the year round to create a mini-garden on your work surface or countertop. Mung beans are a particular favourite for their nutty flavour and delicate texture, but this technique also works to sprout any grain, seed or bean; it's exactly the same process. I like to add mung bean sprouts to a salad or sandwich, or eat them hot in Beansprout and Noodle Chaos (page 196).

MAKES 1 × 1-LITRE (35fl oz) JAR

PREPARATION TIME 4 DAYS

100g (3½oz/½ cup) dried mung beans

EQUIPMENT NEEDED

1 large glass jar (like those in an old-fashioned sweet or candy shop)

1 small piece of muslin (cheesecloth), to cover the neck of the jar

1 rubber band

OPTIONS AND VARIATIONS

To give your children a close-up view of how seeds germinate, soak a selection of dried beans overnight. In the morning, rinse them and lay them on a folded paper towel. Put the paper towel on a saucer and soak it with water. Leave the beans out in the open or cover them with an upturned drinking glass when no one is studying them. Make sure that the towel remains damp and have a magnifying glass nearby, so that changes can be closely observed. Try this with a couple of each of brown lentils, chickpeas (garbanzo beans), kidney beans, adzuki beans, and black-eyed beans (peas).

Rinse the dried beans and tip them into the jar. Add 500ml (17fl oz/2 cups) cold water and leave them to soak overnight.

The next morning, drain away the soaking water. Add more water to the jar to rinse the beans – give them a good swirl – then drain off that water and cover the neck of the jar with the piece of muslin, holding it in place with the rubber band. Leave in natural light at room temperature all day.

In the evening, rinse the beans again and drain them again. (You can leave the muslin in place or remove it during this process.)

Rest the jar on its side with the beans spread out along its length. Keep the jar at room temperature and out of direct sunlight.

Repeat the rinsing and draining every morning and evening for another 2–3 days until the sprouts are about 3cm (1¼in) long.

The sprouts are now ready to be eaten. Tip them out of the jar into a colander. Rinse and drain, and store in the refrigerator in a covered container. This will slow but not stop their growth: they will keep well for about a week, provided you rinse and drain them each day and return them to the refrigerator.

✳ **SPROUTING CHANGES** Soaking seeds, grains or beans before you cook them rehydrates them, causing them to swell, and can reduce their phytic acid content. Phytic acid is sometimes beneficial, but it also can 'bind' with mineral nutrients, making them unavailable to you. Soaking signals to the bean that it is time to sprout, which changes the chemistry of the bean. Because the seed is preparing to grow, it starts to convert its starches, proteins and fats. Usually, they become easier for you to digest and assimilate. Vitamins and enzymes are also produced that add to the bean's nutrient profile.

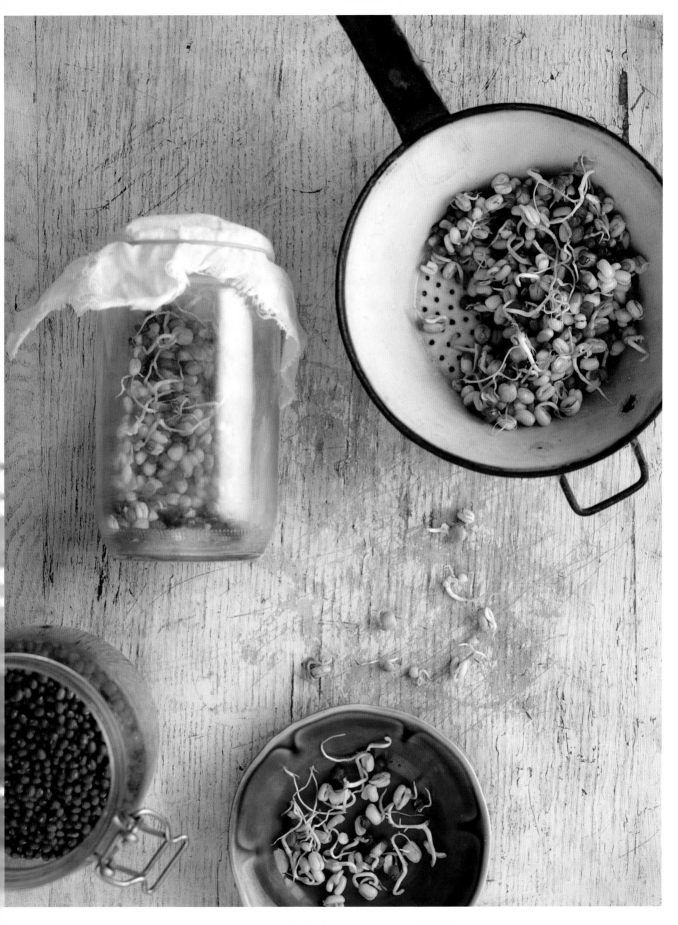

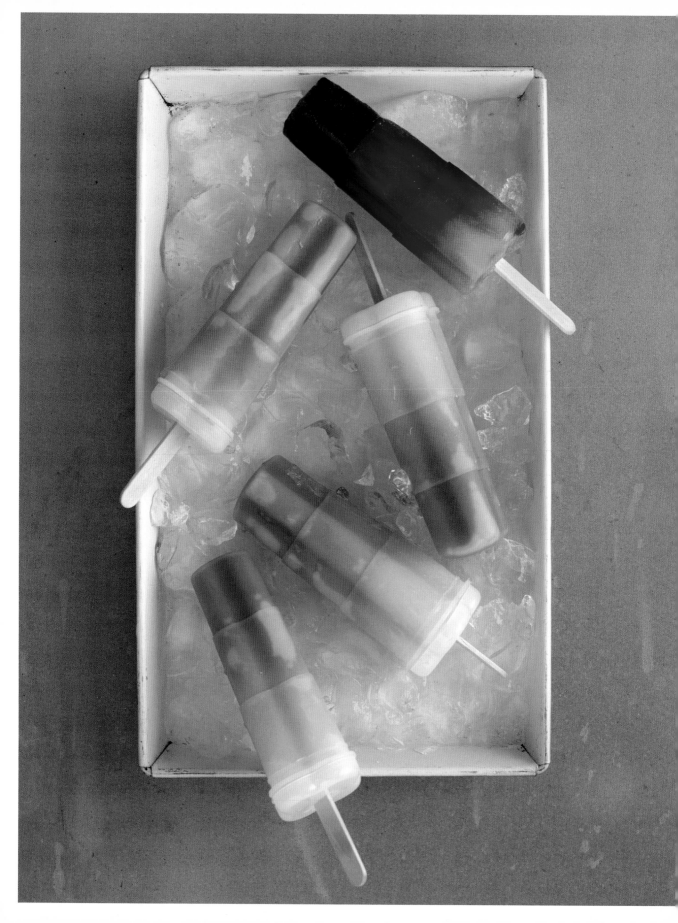

EPIC ICE LOLLIES

Use these fun and colourful iced treats to sneak a little naturally sweet nutritional goodness into family members. Buy organic juices of carrot, beetroot (beet) and apple – or, if you have a juicer or blender, make these juices yourself (in which case, you might like to add a nugget of fresh ginger to the juicer to give extra tang). Increase or decrease the number of layers in your lollies depending on the juices you have – and the time you and your family wish to spend on this edible project. One thing to note: beetroot juice can stain cotton clothing. Your children will be too busy enjoying their lollies and showing off their red tongues and won't mind one bit – but you might!

MAKES 4 LOLLIES (POPSICLES)

PREPARATION TIME 10 MINUTES
+ FREEZING

120ml (4fl oz/½ cup) apple juice

120ml (4fl oz/½ cup) beetroot (beet) juice

120ml (4fl oz/½ cup) carrot juice

OPTIONS AND VARIATIONS

For non-striped lollies, simply mix 3 tablespoons apple juice with the same amount of either beetroot or carrot juice, to give a total of 90ml (3fl oz) of liquid for each lolly. Pour into a lolly (popsicle) mould and freeze. Cordials, either homemade or purchased, can be diluted with water or other juices: for instance, use 60ml (2fl oz/¼ cup) elderflower cordial diluted with 2 tablespoons water to make one highly flavoured elderflower lolly. Fill a lolly mould with some Iced Midsummer Tisane (page 82) to create a lolly with extra zing.

For stripy lollies (popsicles), freeze the juices in stages. Pour about 30ml (1fl oz) of one of the juices – whichever you fancy – into each lolly mould, and leave to freeze for about 1 hour until set.

Add 30ml (1fl oz) of a different coloured juice to each mould for the next layer, and leave to freeze for another hour.

Add 30ml (1fl oz) of the third juice for the final layer, and freeze until ready to eat. To serve, run a little warm water over the outside of the moulds to release the lollies.

EPIC CUBES Add these tangy ice cubes to sparkling water for an instant treat, or use them to cool the refreshing Iced Midsummer Tisane (page 82). Simply pour the juice of 2 lemons and 3 limes into an ice-cube tray. Pop the tray in the freezer and wait! You'll be able to tell by the colour which is lemon and which is lime. You can also use the juice of oranges and grapefruit. Any leftover halves of citrus fruit, or small amounts of apple, carrot or beetroot juice, can be turned into refreshing Epic Cubes.

ICED MIDSUMMER TISANE

There is not a trace of caffeine in this refreshing infusion, but the herbs and spices deliver a delicious, uplifting 'hit'. Each of them has a history of use as a tonic to help strengthen the immune system: brought together in one drink, they give a pleasantly stimulating effect. You'll need a batch of zesty Epic Cubes (page 81) underway in your freezer before you make this (try to make sure that each serving gets at least one pair of lemon and lime cubes). Those who prefer a sweeter drink can stir a little barley malt syrup into their serving.

Put the lemon balm, ginger, fennel seeds, cloves and cayenne into a large teapot or nonreactive pan, and pour over 1 litre (35fl oz/4 cups) boiling water. Cover and set aside to cool.

Strain the tea into a large jug (pitcher), and chill. Just before serving, add the Epic Cubes.

MAKES 1 LITRE (4 CUPS)

PREPARATION TIME 1 HOUR

1 small handful of fresh lemon balm leaves

4 thin slices of fresh ginger

1 tablespoon fennel seeds

6 whole cloves

¼ teaspoon cayenne pepper

1 ice tray of Epic Cubes (page 81)

OPTIONS AND VARIATIONS

Use fresh lemon mint instead of the lemon balm, if you can find it!

TAHINI LEMON WHIP

Use this simple, refreshing whip as a spread, a dressing or a topping for baked potato. I like the texture to be fluffy and light, rather than runny. It can be served over warm or hot dishes, or kept chilled for serving with cold foods. Delicious as a dip with a Crudité Platter (page 239) or with a slice of Rosemary Twist (page 164).

MAKES ABOUT 250ml (1 CUP)

PREPARATION TIME 15 MINUTES

100ml (3½fl oz/scant ½ cup) tahini

Juice of 1 lemon

2 garlic cloves, crushed

Pinch of salt

OPTIONS AND VARIATIONS

For extra spiciness, add ¼ teaspoon of cayenne pepper. Stir in 2 tablespoons chopped fresh coriander leaves.

Whisk together all the ingredients to give a custard-like texture. Set aside for 5 minutes. If you want a lighter texture, add 50ml (1½fl oz) cold water or some more lemon juice, and whisk again.

✱ **WHOLE TAHINI** is a 'butter' made from whole sesame seeds. It is darker than ordinary tahini, which is a pale tan colour. Try both to see which you enjoy the most, but note that the whole form is richer in minerals and protein. Both forms emulsify with liquids such as lemon juice and water. (This is what thickens the whip and why, after it is put aside for a short time, you might wish to add more liquid for the consistency you desire).

✱ I found this dish especially nutritious when I was breastfeeding. It seemed to fortify the milk at about month three and really gave me a boost, too. I used toasted pitta bread to dip into the whip, often with a plate of pickles on the side, a combination that worked surprisingly well.

OLD-FASHIONED SEED CAKE

Caraway always imparts a fresh flavour. Here it combines with the slight sweetness of candied citrus peel. As with other bakes in this book, vinegar is used to activate the baking powder, to help make the cake rise. The aim is to keep the two components apart until the very last moment, and then to get the cake into the preheated oven quickly. You need have to have everything ready and stir the batter only briefly, but it's worth the slight last-minute rush for a nicely risen cake. As it's not iced, you can serve slightly warm slices – usually straight into eagerly awaiting hands! If they can bear to wait for a plate, this is delicious served with a spoonful of marmalade or Plum Butter (page 45).

MAKES 1 SQUARE OR LOAF CAKE

PREPARATION TIME 45 MINUTES

125g (4½oz) coconut oil, plus extra for greasing the pan

140ml (4½fl oz/½ cup plus 1 tablespoon) barley malt syrup

125g (4½oz/⅔ cup, lightly packed) soft light brown sugar

200ml (7fl oz/scant 1 cup) plant milk

1 tablespoon apple cider vinegar

250g (9oz/1⅔ cups) plain (all-purpose) or wholemeal (whole-wheat) flour

100g (3½oz) mixed candied citrus peel

4 teaspoons caraway seeds

2 teaspoons baking powder

½ teaspoon ground cinnamon

¼ teaspoon ground nutmeg

OPTIONS AND VARIATIONS

Use half-and-half plain (all-purpose) and wholemeal (whole-wheat) flours. Add ½ teaspoon ground ginger to the dry mixture.

Preheat the oven to 200°C (400°F), and grease a 20cm (8in) square cake pan or 900g (2lb) loaf pan with coconut oil.

Melt the 125g (4½oz) coconut oil over a low heat and whisk in the syrup. Dissolve the sugar in the plant milk in a measuring jug (large measuring cup), then whisk in the oil and syrup. Add the vinegar and stir briefly. Set aside to cool slightly.

Mix together the flour, candied peel, caraway seeds, baking powder, cinnamon and nutmeg in a large bowl.

Working swiftly now, tip the wet mixture into the dry ingredients and stir as briefly as possible, while ensuring that everything is thoroughly and evenly mixed. Pour the batter into the prepared cake pan, spread it out and level the top; bake for 5 minutes. Reduce the oven temperature to 180°C (350°F), and bake for a further 20–25 minutes until risen and golden, and a skewer or the tip of a sharp knife inserted into the centre comes out clean.

Let the cooked cake rest in the pan for 10 minutes, before turning it out onto a wire rack to cool before serving.

EGG ALTERNATIVES Eggs are not part of the vegan diet, so here are some handy plant-based alternatives for use in baking:

✷ 60ml (2fl oz/¼ cup) plant milk or water will supply the moisture of 1 egg

✷ 1 tablespoon tahini whisked into 60ml (2fl oz/¼ cup) of liquid will add a binding effect

✷ 1 tablespoon lemon juice or apple cider vinegar, combined with 1 teaspoon bicarbonate of soda (baking soda), adds the lightness of 1 egg, especially when stirred together at the last moment

✷ 70ml (2¼fl oz) apple sauce or Apple Butter (page 43) will help to bind and lighten as for 1 egg

✷ 50g (1¾oz) plain tofu puréed with 2 tablespoons of liquid will bind and lighten as for 1 egg

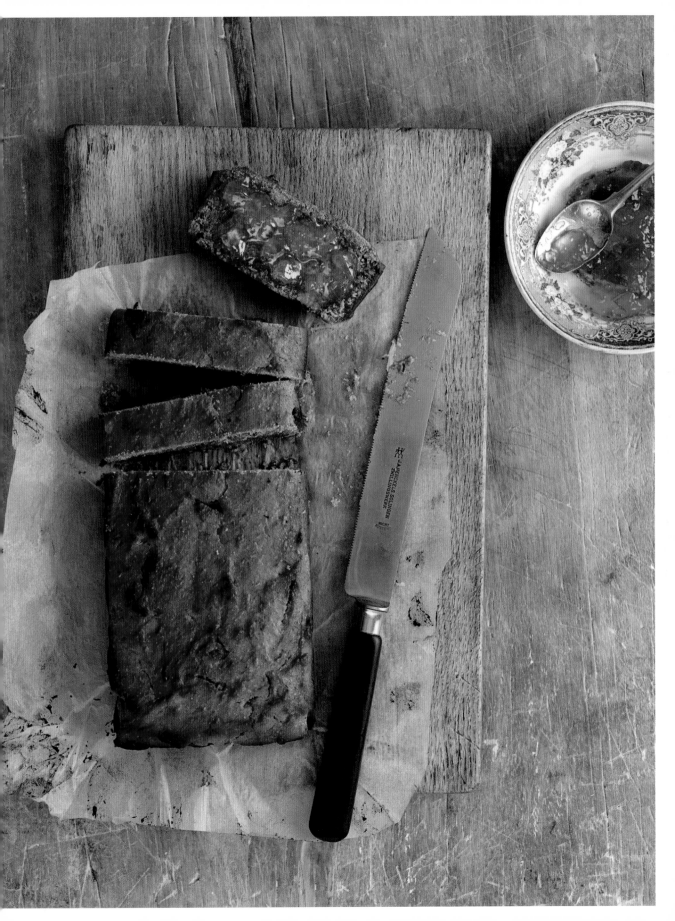

ROASTED SEED MIXTURE

I associate this treat with winter evenings because it was a favourite when our teenagers arrived home, out of the dark and cold. It is perfect for snacks and packed lunches at any time of year and especially comforting when unexpected guests arrive. Then the aroma and popping sound create anticipation and a sense of welcome. Take care to serve the mixture warm but not hot, especially if it is to be nibbled as a snack. The seeds hold the heat and can burn your mouth if eaten too soon. Sprinkle over salads or a serving of freshly cooked grains, such as Three-Grain Risotto (page 184).

SERVES 4

PREPARATION TIME 15 MINUTES

100g (3½oz/1 cup) flaked almonds

150g (5½oz/1 cup) shelled pumpkin seeds (pepitas)

225g (8oz/1½ cups) shelled sunflower seeds

1 tablespoon tamari

OPTIONS AND VARIATIONS

Add 75g (2½oz/½ cup) pine nuts to the mixture as it is cooling in the pan: do not roast the pine nuts; simply stir them into the hot seeds.

Warm a large frying pan (skillet) over a medium heat. Add the almonds and the pumpkin and sunflower seeds, and stir them as they roast. It is important to tend them carefully, as they can burn easily. They are ready when you can see a little browning on some of them – and when you hear them start to pop!

Remove the pan from the heat, and keep stirring the mixture as you drizzle the tamari over the seeds and nuts. The residual heat of the pan will help to distribute the tamari.

Keep stirring for a minute or so, to ensure that the seeds are nicely coated with the tamari and do not clump together.

Tip out the seeds onto a plate to cool a little, before serving individual portions in small bowls.

✳ **ROASTING NUTS AND SEEDS** Having made this mixture, I took to roasting other nuts in the same way. I found that roasting them with no additional oil allowed flavours to emerge that I hadn't noticed before. Raw cashews brown nicely in a hot pan, when stirred almost constantly, and are excellent over stir-fried noodles. I roast walnuts in this way, too, and find their flavour greatly intensified. I keep my batches of roasted nuts and seeds to a quantity that I know will be eaten within 24 hours because I've noticed that they lose their flavour if left for much longer. This is one mixture that is best made fresh, and not stored.

SEEDED SPELT BREAD

Spelt is an ancestor of modern wheat and is used in the same way, but it has a different nutrient profile. It can be mixed with other wheat flours, whether white or wholemeal (whole-wheat), but is great all by itself, as I hope this bread will prove. Serve it, sliced and toasted, and spread with Herb and Onion Bean Butter (page 71), or use it to make a Kohlrabi and Cucumber Sandwich (page 123).

MAKES 2 LOAVES

PREPARATION TIME 3 HOURS +

4 HOURS SOAKING

1 tablespoon whole flaxseeds (linseeds)

1 teaspoon granulated sugar

1 × 8g sachet or 2 teaspoons dried yeast

1kg (2¼lb) wholemeal (wholegrain) spelt flour

3 tablespoons extra virgin olive oil

OPTIONS AND VARIATIONS

For a darker, richly flavoured loaf, dissolve 1 tablespoon blackstrap molasses in 250ml (9fl oz/1 cup) warm water, and mix the sugar and yeast in a separate jug (large measuring cup) with another 250ml (9fl oz/1 cup) warm water. Add them to flour at the same time.

Measure the flaxseeds into a small bowl and add 3 tablespoons cold water. Cover the bowl and leave the seeds to soak for at least 4 hours, or preferably overnight.

When the seeds are ready, measure 500ml (17fl oz/2 cups) warm water into a measuring jug (large measuring cup), and dissolve the sugar in it. Add the yeast, stir well and set the jug aside in a warm place for 5–10 minutes until the mixture begins to froth.

Put the flour in a bowl. Measure out an extra 200ml (7fl oz/scant 1 cup) warm water and keep it close to hand.

When the yeast mixture is frothy, pour it into the flour. Add the olive oil and soaked flaxseeds, including their soaking water (which will be slightly gel-like). Use a wooden spoon to stir the liquids into the flour. When this begins to become difficult, use your hands.

Begin to knead the dough, adding some of the extra water if needed – you're aiming for a dough that is firm and not sticky. Knead the dough for at least 5 minutes. Shape the dough into a ball and leave it in the bowl, covered with a cloth, in a warm place to rise. After about 1 hour, it should have risen to roughly double its original size.

Lightly oil two 900g (2lb) loaf pans. When the dough has risen, rub a little oil on your hands and knead the dough again for 2 minutes. Divide the dough in half and shape into two loaves. Put one in each loaf pan, cover with a cloth and leave to rise again for about 1 hour.

Preheat the oven to 250°C (500°F).

Bake the loaves in the oven for 5 minutes, then reduce the oven temperature to 180°C (350°F) and bake for a further 25–30 minutes until golden brown on top. Turn out the loaves and tap them on the bottom – if they are cooked, they will sound hollow. Turn the loaves onto a wire rack to cool.

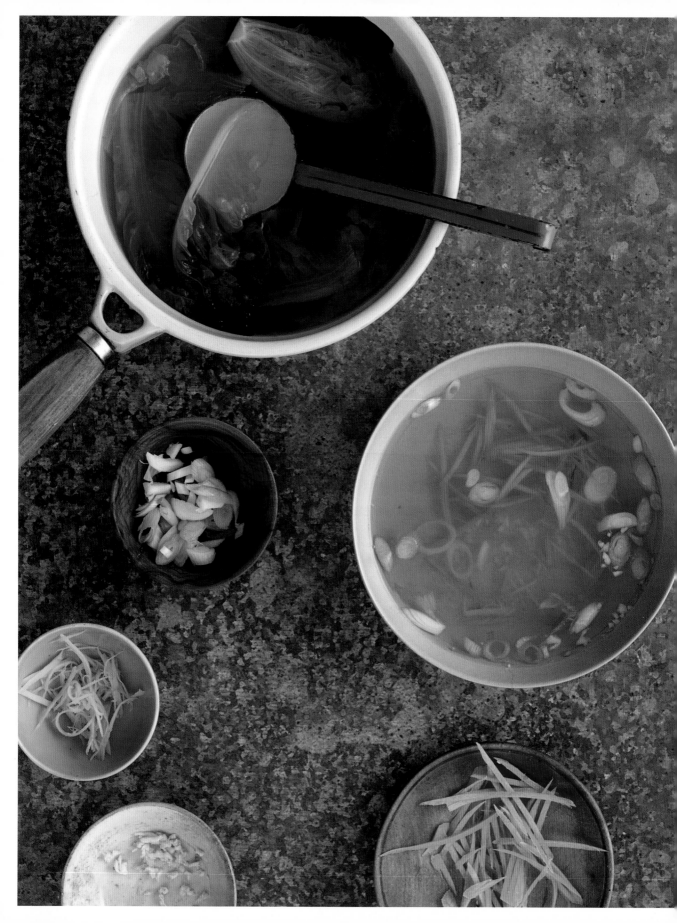

LETTUCE AND GINGER BROTH

When your temperature is up and you start to feel your bones ache, try this broth. It's excellent for flu-like symptoms as well as that late-in-the-day feeling of exhaustion or a yearning to be warm. Don't stop at just one bowlful: finish the batch within 24 hours, and see if you feel better. For extra savour, add a sprinkle of tamari at the last moment.

MAKES 4 BOWLFULS

PREPARATION TIME 30 MINUTES

1 whole cos (romaine) lettuce

10cm (4in) strip of kombu, rinsed

FOR EACH BOWLFUL

3 tablespoons grated carrot

1 tablespoon grated ginger

1 spring onion (scallion), finely sliced

1 garlic clove, finely chopped

OPTIONS AND VARIATIONS

To make the broth even more warming, add a pinch of cayenne pepper or ground nutmeg to your soup bowl.

Bring 2 litres (70fl oz/8 cups) water to the boil in a large stockpot or saucepan.

Trim the lettuce, slicing through about 3cm (1¼in) from the root end to separate the leaves. Rinse the leaves and add them to the boiling water. Stir so that the leaves are immersed. Add the kombu, cover the pan, reduce the heat and simmer for 20 minutes.

Put a serving of the prepared carrot, ginger, onion and garlic in your bowl(s). Ladle over the hot broth (leaving the lettuce leaves behind in the pot of broth). Stir the contents of the soup bowl, and leave to steep until cool enough to eat.

Leave the lettuce leaves and kombu in the broth until the broth has cooled, then discard them. That way, all the goodness is drawn into the broth. Reheat the broth as needed and ladle it, hot, over bowlfuls of the fresh ingredients.

RICE, RADISH AND SPICE SALAD

When you need a little something that is light yet filling, try this salad. It has a zesty flavour, and the variety of fresh ingredients ensures great nutrition, too. It improves in flavour if it is covered and allowed to stand, which makes it an excellent meal to prepare ahead – I find it is also improved by a period of chilling. Make it and store it in the refrigerator overnight. It is easy to pack and carry to work or school the next day. Use any type of rice, including red rice, wild rice or basmati rice. I like to serve the salad with Margarita Yogurt Dip (see below).

Combine all of the ingredients in a large bowl. Mix well, and leave to stand for 1 hour if possible, or chill until ready to serve.

MARGARITA YOGURT DIP Yogurt can take the heat from spices such as chillies, which is why you'll often find it served as a 'side' to spicy dishes – to help you survive the meal! Serve this as a cooling and refreshing dip with crudités, pitta bread or corn chips, and it makes a delicious dressing for a plate of sliced, fresh tomatoes, too. I enjoy its blend of pungent and slightly sour flavours. Add a dollop to Ruby Root Soup (page 248). And it is excellent served beside Simple Red Lentil Dhal (page 201). In a serving bowl, stir together 300g (10½oz/1¼ cups) plain, unsweetened soya yogurt, 1 finely chopped small red onion, 1 finely chopped small cucumber, 3 tablespoons each of finely chopped fresh basil and coriander (cilantro) leaves, and a pinch of salt. Stir well, cover and chill well before serving. You can add ¼ teaspoon crushed caraway or dill seed as an optional extra.

✷ **UME SHISO SEASONING** is a Japanese product that is available from some grocers and health food stores, as well as by online purchase. It is made from plum vinegar and coloured a beautiful pink by shiso leaves, which can be bought from farmers' markets in the spring and summer. Shiso leaves are also excellent in salads, to include in a batch of fresh pickles or to cook with summer greens.

SERVES 4
PREPARATION TIME 15 MINUTES

300g (10½oz/about 1⅓ cups) cooked rice of any sort

6 radishes, chopped

2 spring onions (scallions), finely chopped

1 medium carrot, grated

40g (1½oz/1¼ cups) fresh rocket (arugula), chopped

A small handful of fresh basil and flat-leaf parsley, chopped

100g (3½oz) firm smoked or seeded tofu, cut into cubes (about ½ cup prepared)

¼ teaspoon ground nutmeg

1 tablespoon extra virgin olive oil

1 teaspoon apple cider vinegar

1 teaspoon ume shiso seasoning

OPTIONS AND VARIATIONS

For a more mellow flavour, use rice wine vinegar instead of the cider vinegar. For added crunch, add 2 tablespoons pine nuts or sunflower seeds. Add 2 tablespoons capers for a fleeting taste sensation.

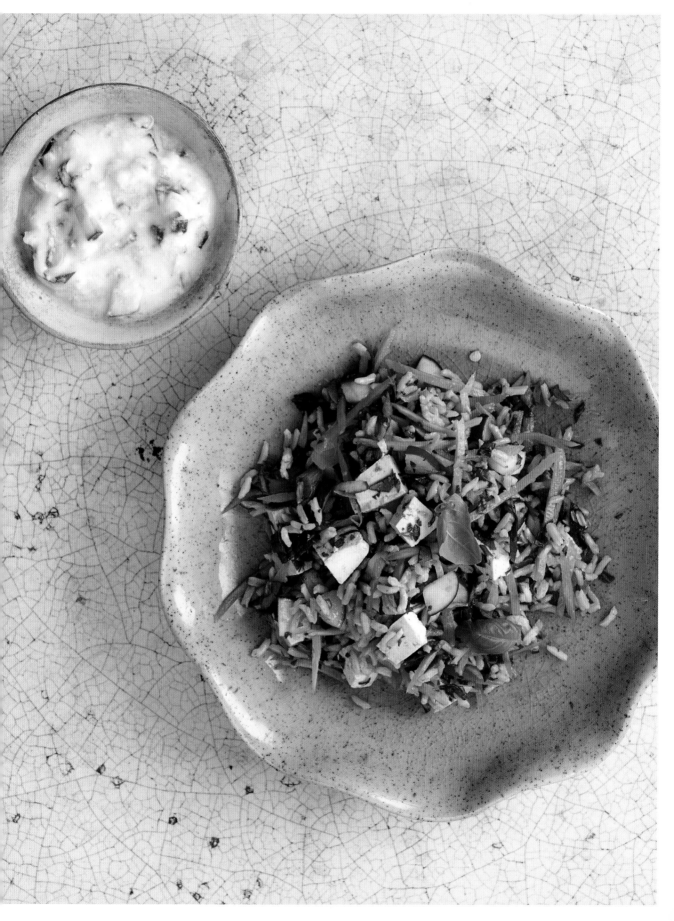

ENTIRELY GREEN SALAD

Escape the monotony of iceberg lettuce and make a tasty salad from the wonderful variety of flavoursome and nutritious leaves that changes with the seasons. Here are some ideas and combinations that you might enjoy experimenting with. For a dressing, less is often more – a drizzle of extra virgin olive oil and rice wine vinegar might be just right. Or, offer a selection: try Velvet Vinaigrette (page 244) or Herb and Garlic Drizzle (page 209).

SERVES 4

PREPARATION TIME 15 MINUTES

BITTER dandelion, endive, chicory, radicchio, crisp lettuce (such as iceberg)

LEMONY sorrel, lemon balm, lemon mint

SWEET peppermint, basil, fennel leaf, cress, chervil, oakleaf lettuce

TANGY baby spinach, shiso, coriander (cilantro)

EARTHY parsley, tarragon, cos (romaine) lettuce, purslane

PEPPERY rocket (arugula), nasturtium leaves, watercress or land cress

PUNGENT wild garlic (ramps), chives, spring onion (scallion) greens

OPTIONS AND VARIATIONS

Add edible flowers such as nasturtium, courgette (zucchini), rose petals or wild garlic (ramps).

Select your 'base' leaf, such as one of the lettuces listed. Shred or tear enough for four servings (about 160g/5½oz, depending on the bulkiness of the leaves and the size of portions you prefer), and add to a large salad bowl.

Select one or two 'companion' leaves from other flavour groups and add these to the salad bowl. In total, these leaves need only comprise half as much salad as the base leaf.

Select very small amounts of one or two more leaves. These will emerge as 'finishing notes' to a mouthful of salad. Occasionally, they will be surprising taste sensations. For instance, you might have quite an earthy base flavour with companion leaves that are peppery and 'finishing notes' from a tablespoon of chopped chives or lemon mint.

Toss the leaves together and taste a forkful without dressing. This will help you to decide what sort of dressing flavour to aim for.

✱ **TO CLEAN AND REVIVE FRESH SALAD GREENS** add 150ml (5fl oz) white or apple cider vinegar to a sinkful of cold water. Add the greens, placing a plate over them to keep them immersed, and soak for 10–15 minutes. Lift from the water and use a salad spinner to remove excess water.

QUICKLY SALAD

I'm as keen as anyone to reduce stress levels and endless rushing, but sometimes we simply have to be quick. Here is a good dose of tasty green herbs and back-garden extras that can be dished up double-quick. Serve as a starter to any pasta dish, or on the plate beside Mediterranean Spiced Rice and Lentils (page 130). I love this salad with a thin drizzle of pomegranate molasses on my portion.

Finely chop the mint, rocket, tomato, spring onions, and courgette, and put them in a bowl. Slice the radishes and add to the bowl. Next, add the basil, olive oil and lemon juice. Season with salt and pepper.

Toss the salad together and serve immediately, or cover and refrigerate for use later the same day – the flavours will develop.

SERVES 4

PREPARATION TIME 10 MINUTES

1 handful of fresh mint leaves

50g (1¾oz/1½ cups) fresh rocket (arugula)

1 medium tomato

2 spring onions (scallions)

1 small courgette (zucchini)

6 medium radishes

2 tablespoons chopped fresh basil

2 tablespoons extra virgin olive oil

Juice of 1 lemon

Salt and pepper, to taste

OPTIONS AND VARIATIONS

For some quick croûtons, toast a slice of Splendid Wholesome Loaf (page 120) so that it is crispy. Cut into cubes, and toss them into the salad at the very last minute.

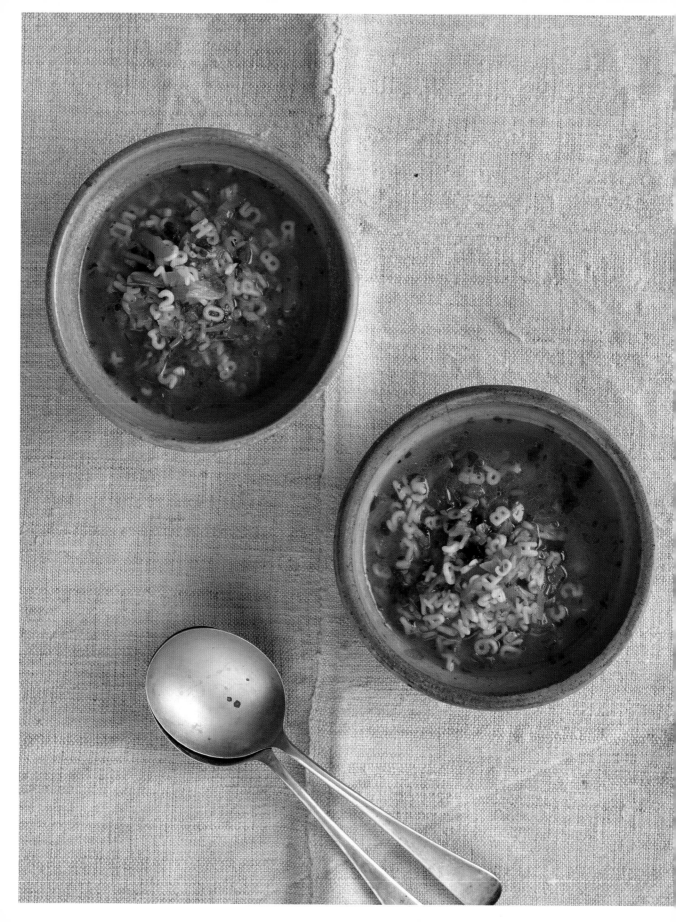

ALPHABET SOUP

No child can resist this, for the fun of the pasta letters. Few adults can resist it either, for the delicate flavour and aroma of the chervil, the other special ingredient in this light springtime soup. Chervil has many common names, including sweet cicely. You can sometimes find it at a farmers' market in spring, or perhaps from a local herb grower. Alphabet pasta cooks very quickly and each letter swells as it cooks. For this reason, in this recipe it is added right at the end of cooking and the pan is immediately removed from the heat. Try to share out the whole panful in one sitting, so that the pasta does not soak up too much of the broth and become waterlogged. Everyone, of any age, will want to spell out a word – maybe on the plate, next to an Avocado Rocket Launch Sandwich (page 123).

SERVES 4
PREPARATION TIME 30 MINUTES

1 tablespoon untoasted sesame oil

8cm (3¼in) strip of kombu, rinsed

1 medium onion, finely chopped

2 garlic cloves, finely chopped

¼ teaspoon black pepper

Pinch of Chinese five-spice

1 medium carrot, grated

50g (1¾oz) fresh chervil, finely chopped

4 tablespoons alphabet pasta

OPTIONS AND VARIATIONS

To make this soup when chervil cannot be found, use chopped celery leaves instead of the chervil. They'll need slightly longer to cook, so add the celery leaves with the grated carrot.

Pour the oil into a saucepan set over a low to medium heat. Add the kombu, onion, garlic, black pepper and five-spice, cover the pan and sauté for 10–12 minutes until the onion is tender.

Add the grated carrots and stir well. Cover the pan and cook for a further 5 minutes. Add the chervil and stir for 1 minute, then add 1 litre (35fl oz/4 cups) water and bring the soup to a low simmer.

Remove the kombu from the pan (if it has not already dissolved) and stir in the alphabet pasta. Cover the pan and remove it from the heat. Set aside for 10 minutes before serving, to allow the pasta to cook in the residual heat.

CHOCOLATE CHIP COOKIES

Start a family tradition! This classic cookie can easily be adapted to suit your tastes and the texture you most enjoy. Follow the recipe for a firm, chocolate-rich cookie that is not too sweet. You can adjust the texture: for a thinner, softer cookie, reduce the quantity of bran by half. Experiment until you find your perfect cookie. For those who can't get enough chocolate, these are excellent with Choc Hotlate (page 171).

Preheat the oven to 200°C (400°F), and lightly oil two baking sheets.

In a measuring jug (large measuring cup), whisk together the sugar, tahini, oil, milk and vanilla extract. In a large bowl, stir together the flour, oat bran, baking powder and chocolate chips.

Pour the wet mixture into the dry mixture, and stir well. Drop portions of the dough onto the baking sheets, and bake for 12–15 minutes until the cookies are golden.

Leave the cookies to cool on their sheets for 5 minutes, before transferring them to a wire rack to cool completely.

MAKES 12 LARGE COOKIES

PREPARATION TIME 45 MINUTES

100g (3½oz/½ cup, lightly packed) soft light brown sugar

140ml (4½fl oz/generous ½ cup) tahini

60ml (2fl oz/¼ cup) untoasted sesame oil, plus extra for brushing the baking sheets

170ml (5½fl oz/⅔ cup) plant milk

1 teaspoon vanilla extract

170g (6oz/scant 1¼ cups) plain (all-purpose) or wholemeal (whole-wheat) flour

2 tablespoons oat bran

2 teaspoons baking powder

200g (7oz/1¼ cups) dark chocolate chips

OPTIONS AND VARIATIONS

Almond milk and coconut milk will add a little hint of their flavour to this recipe. If you use almond milk, you might like to use almond extract in place of the vanilla.

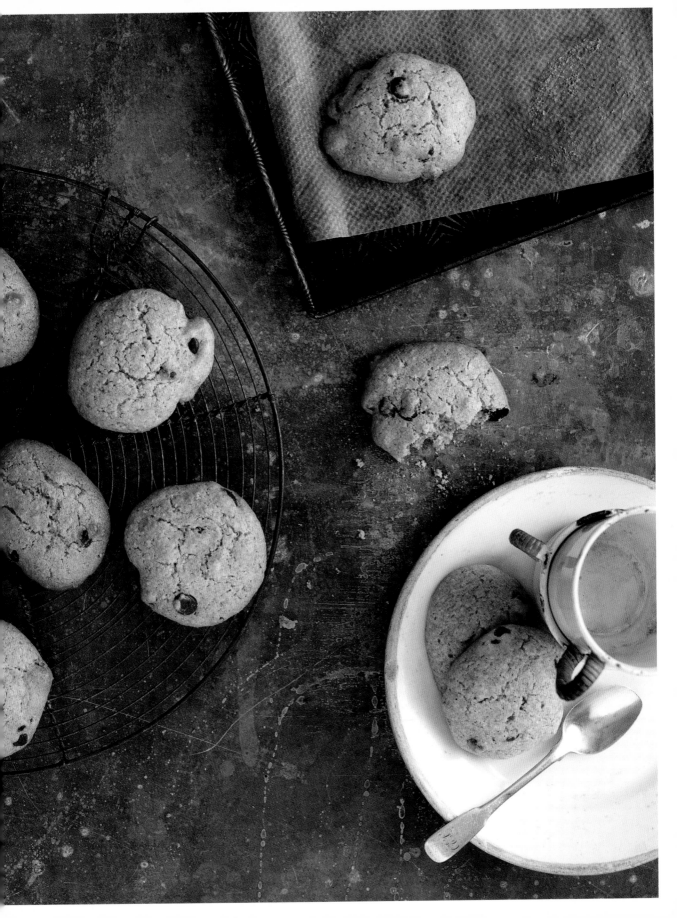

LUNCH

EGG SALAD LOOKALIKE SANDWICH

It was never my intention to make this a lookalike, but more than one person has commented on its resemblance to an egg mayonnaise sandwich, so the name has stuck. It is delicious – and not an egg included! Make two, and sip a glass of Iced Midsummer Tisane (page 82) between bites.

Spread the slices of bread with bean butter, followed by a thin layer of mustard. In a small bowl, mix together the cheese, carrot, onion and mayonnaise. Spread this onto one slice of bread, top with the other slice of bread, and serve.

MAKES 1 SANDWICH

PREPARATION TIME 10 MINUTES

2 slices of fresh bread

2 tablespoons Herb and Onion Bean Butter (page 71)

1 teaspoon favourite mustard

50g (1¾oz/about ⅓ cup) grated vegan cheese

½ small carrot, grated

1 spring onion (scallion), finely chopped

2 tablespoons vegan mayonnaise or Tofu-Mayo (see right)

OPTIONS AND VARIATIONS

A tablespoon of grated turnip adds a tangy taste sensation to the filling, or add a splash of hot sauce or Tabasco. You can add some lettuce, cucumber and tomato, but bear in mind that the filling is likely to slide: take care not to end up with vegan egg salad in your lap! Fill a baguette instead of sliced bread.

TOFU-MAYO There are many brands of vegan mayonnaise available, so this is possibly unnecessary – and not quite mayonnaise! But when it's midnight, the shops are shut and you need something like mayo … you might want to give this a try. Using a fork, mash together 60g (2oz) firm, plain tofu and 1 teaspoon Dijon mustard in a small bowl. Mix 60ml (2fl oz/¼ cup) extra virgin olive oil with 2 tablespoons tahini and beat this mixture, a little at a time, into the tofu mixture. After each addition, add a little lemon or lime juice. Continue in this way, adjusting for consistency and flavour. Season to taste with a little salt, stir well, and transfer the mixture into a jar with a tight-fitting lid. Store in the refrigerator. Add it to sandwiches, such as the one above or Kohlrabi and Cucumber Sandwich (page 123), or spoon a little over salads or a baked potato.

POLENTA WITH GARDEN GARLAND

Maize, or sweetcorn, is one of the foods that has sustained humans since the Neolithic Revolution. Polenta is the ground kernel, traditionally cooked into a porridge. In this recipe, the polenta undergoes a simple two-part preparation, before being surrounded by fresh treasures from the garden. When I eat this, I try to make sure each forkful includes a bit of sliced polenta and some of the vegetables. Serve with a little Almond, Lime and Fresh Herb Pesto (page 176) or Sweetcorn and Pepper Relish (page 134) on each plate.

SERVES 4

PREPARATION TIME 45 MINUTES

250g (9oz/1⅓ cups) coarse polenta

1 tablespoon untoasted sesame oil

FOR THE GARDEN GARLAND

160g (5¾oz) slender stalks of purple sprouting or Tenderstem broccoli

200g (7oz) asparagus

120g (4oz/about 1 cup) French (string) beans, trimmed

1 medium tomato, chopped

50g (1¾oz/1½ cups) fresh rocket (arugula), finely chopped

1 spring onion (scallion), finely chopped

1 lemon, quartered

1 tablespoon chopped fresh basil

A little extra virgin olive oil for dressing

Salt and pepper, to taste

OPTIONS AND VARIATIONS

Grill vegetables such as baby courgettes (zucchini) or sweet pepper (capsicum) slices and add to the garland.

Bring 1 litre (35fl oz/4 cups) water to the boil in a saucepan. Add a pinch of salt and pour the polenta flour into the pan. Stir well with a wooden spoon or spurtle. Keep the pan over a low to medium heat and keep stirring as the cornmeal thickens, for 20–30 minutes.

Dampen a large baking sheet with cold water, then spread the cooked polenta over it to an even thickness of about 2cm (¾in). You will have to work quickly – it helps to have a dampened spoon or table knife for the spreading. Set the polenta aside to cool completely.

To prepare the garden garland, pour water into a large saucepan to a depth of 4cm (1½in). Fit a steaming basket over the water and set the pan over a medium heat. Put the broccoli, asparagus and beans into the steaming basket and cover the pan. Steam for 10 minutes until the greens are just tender. Arrange on individual plates.

Mix together the tomato, rocket and spring onion in a bowl. Season with salt and pepper, and arrange on the individual plates. Dress with a little olive oil and a squeeze of fresh lemon.

To finish the polenta, pour the sesame oil into a frying pan set over a medium heat. Slice the cold polenta into an even number of pieces and lightly fry the slices for 2–3 minutes on each side until golden and slightly crisp. Arrange slices of fried polenta on the individual plates, sprinkle with fresh basil and serve.

✱ **VERSATILE POLENTA** Make a double batch of polenta and store unfried slices in the refrigerator to eat the next day, perhaps with a little Avocado Press (page 72) or Apple Butter (page 43).

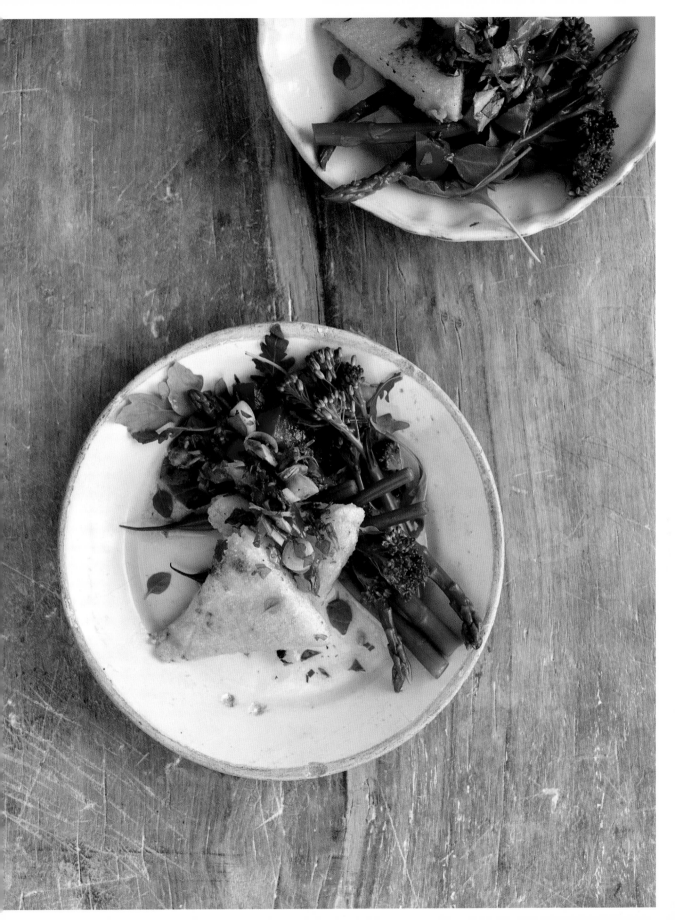

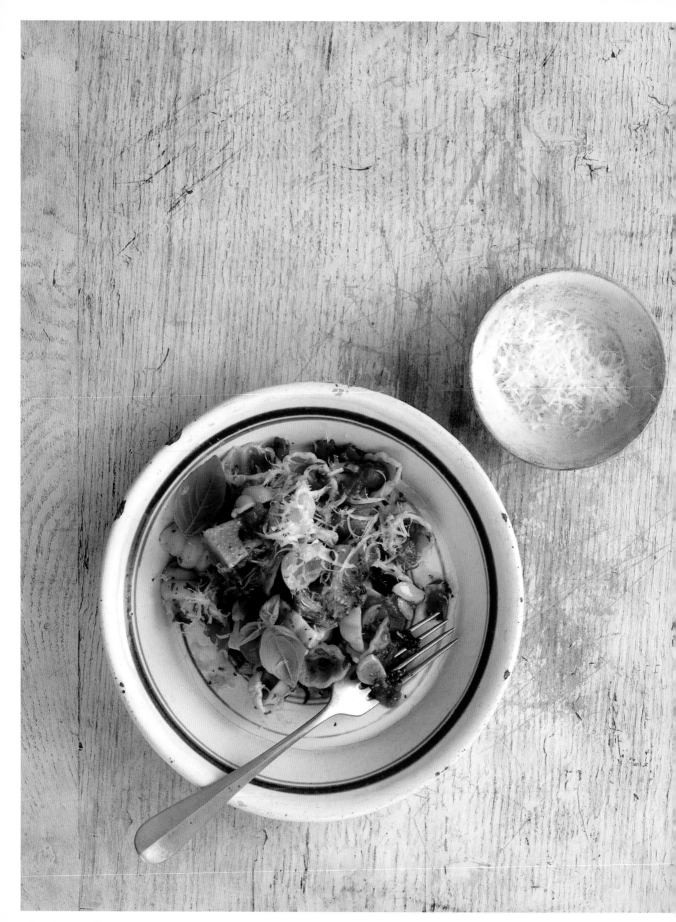

GARLIC AND ARTICHOKE CONCHIGLIE

There is some controversy over whether you should serve your sauce over your pasta, or stir it into your pasta ... I tend to make an executive decision! The garlic in this dish takes on a very mellow tone so, although there is a lot of it, don't worry about it being antisocial. I love to serve a small bowl of fresh Sprouted Mung Beans (page 78) on the side: their clean and crispy influence somehow heightens my enjoyment of the pasta.

SERVES 4

PREPARATION TIME 40 MINUTES

1 tablespoon untoasted sesame oil

1 whole garlic bulb, cloves separated and halved from base to tip

6 large stalks fresh parsley, leaves picked and finely chopped

2 teaspoons dried basil

2 medium tomatoes, chopped

8–10 cooked artichoke hearts, quartered

500g (1lb 2oz) conchiglie pasta

4 tablespoons chopped fresh basil

A little extra virgin olive oil for drizzling

Salt and pepper, to taste

OPTIONS AND VARIATIONS

Add half a dozen cooked white beans to each portion.

Pour the oil into a large saucepan set over a low to medium heat.

Add the garlic and parsley, and sauté, covered, for 5 minutes. Add the dried basil, tomatoes and artichokes. Stir well and cover the pan. Reduce the heat and cook for 10 minutes, stirring once or twice in that time.

Meanwhile, set a large pan of water over a high heat and bring to the boil. Add the pasta and cook according to the instructions on the packet, until just tender.

Drain the pasta and divide it among four bowls. Ladle a portion of the sauce over each bowl of pasta. Sprinkle with the fresh basil, season with salt and pepper, and drizzle a little olive oil over each portion just before serving.

FRESH BORLOTTI BEAN SALAD

If you're lucky enough to find these luscious variegated beans in their polka-dot pods at the end of summer, buy them and make this salad: they are exquisite when fresh. I always try to have them as often as I can during their short season. Get everyone to help with shelling the beans and this dish will be very quickly prepared. This salad is ideal for a buffet beside other seasonal treats such as Entirely Green Salad (page 92) or Sauteed Tatsoi in Black Sesame (page 112).

SERVES 4

PREPARATION TIME 25 MINUTES

1kg (2¼lb) fresh borlotti beans in their pods, shelled and rinsed

50g (1¾oz/1½ cups) fresh rocket (arugula), chopped

25g (1oz/½ cup) chopped fresh basil

1 tablespoon chopped fresh mint

2 spring onions (scallions), finely chopped

2 garlic cloves, finely chopped

1 medium tomato, chopped

Salt and pepper, to taste

OPTIONS AND VARIATIONS

Add 1 tablespoon chopped fresh lemon balm to the other greens. Leave this salad dressed in its natural juices, or drizzle a tiny amount of extra virgin olive oil over your portion followed by a teaspoon of freshly squeezed lemon or lime juice.

Bring some water to the boil in a saucepan and add the shelled beans. Cover the pan, reduce the heat and leave the beans to cook for about 10 minutes at a gentle simmer until they are tender.

Meanwhile, combine the rocket, basil, mint, spring onions, garlic and tomato in a serving bowl. Season with salt and pepper, and stir well. The salt will draw the juices out of the tomato, and this will form a little dressing.

When the beans are ready, drain them thoroughly and add them to the salad. Stir well and leave the salad to stand for a few minutes before serving, to allow the flavours to blend.

✳ **BORLOTTI BEANS** are sometimes offered for sale in their pods weeks after they have been harvested. You'll be able to tell: the pods will look shrivelled and be opening slightly. The beans inside will still be delicious, but will have begun to dry. Remove them from their pods and soak them in cold water for 30 minutes before cooking as described above. This will begin to rehydrate them and will shorten the cooking time.

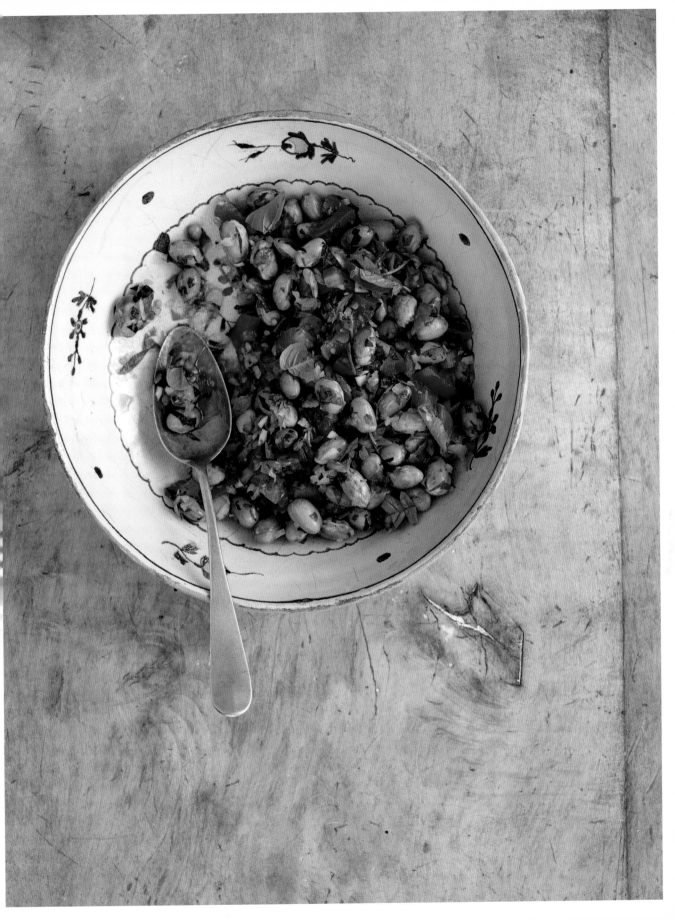

BEAN AND BARLEY SOUP

It's impossible to feel hungry or cold after a bowlful of this soup. Serve it on winter evenings or rainy autumn (fall) days when the wind and chill seems to steal your warmth. Put a fresh loaf of Four-Day Sourdough Bread (page 118) on the table and a wedge of Mung Bean Pâté (page 77) to complete the meal.

SERVES 4

PREPARATION TIME 1 HOUR

50g (1¾oz/scant ⅓ cup) pot (hulled) barley, rinsed

1 tablespoon untoasted sesame oil

2 leeks, trimmed and chopped

2 large onions, chopped

1 teaspoon vegan bouillon powder

½ teaspoon dried basil

½ teaspoon dried oregano

½ teaspoon black pepper

¼ teaspoon Chinese five-spice

¼ teaspoon ground nutmeg

1 litre (35fl oz/4 cups) vegetable stock or water

300g (10½oz/about 2 cups) cooked butter (lima) beans (see How to Cook Beans, page 64)

OPTIONS AND VARIATIONS

Use a 10cm (4in) strip of kombu, rinsed, instead of the bouillon powder. Add this after you have puréed the soup and leave it in until ready to serve.

Put the rinsed barley in a bowl and cover with cold water. Leave to soak for at least 1 hour (and no more than 12).

Pour the oil into a large stockpot or saucepan. Add the leeks and onions, cover the pan and cook over a medium heat for 15 minutes until the onions have softened and released their juices. Add the bouillon, herbs and spices, and stir well. Add 750ml (26fl oz/3 cups) of the stock or water, and use a hand-held blender to purée the mixture.

Drain and rinse the soaked barley and add it to the pan. Stir well, cover the pan and cook over a low to medium heat for 35 minutes.

Add the remaining 250ml (9fl oz/1 cup) stock and the cooked beans; stir well. If you want to eat the soup immediately, bring it to a low simmer and serve. If you have time, however, the soup's flavour will be enhanced by being left to stand for about 8 hours. I tend to make this in the morning and have it for the evening meal.

✻ **POT (HULLED) BARLEY** is almost a whole grain: most of its bran, all but the outermost hull, is still intact. Pearl barley is shiny white by comparison because all of its bran has been removed. Pot barley has a lovely creamy, golden colour when cooked, with flashes of its white centre peeping out through the bran coating. It's rich in soluble and insoluble fibre, B vitamins and a variety of minerals, too. Barley is another of those grains that has been cultivated by humans since ancient times.

CHESTNUT AND CELERIAC SOUP

It's not always clear what brings ingredients together in a dish. Inspiration for this soup struck when, carrying a giant celeriac (celery root) home from the farmers' market, I stopped to sample a freshly roasted chestnut. If you can find them, roast a dozen sweet chestnuts in the oven and crumble two or three of them over each portion of this soup. Alternatively, garnish with a single curl of sweet red pepper. I've found that this soup goes especially well with an Egg Salad Lookalike Sandwich (page 99).

SERVES 4

PREPARATION TIME 40 MINUTES

1 tablespoon untoasted sesame oil

400g (14oz) chopped celeriac (celery root)

2 celery stalks, chopped

2 large onions, finely chopped

1 red sweet pepper (capsicum), deseeded and chopped

½ teaspoon paprika

1 litre (35fl oz/4 cups) vegetable stock or water

2 tablespoons chestnut purée

Salt and pepper, to taste

OPTIONS AND VARIATIONS

If you prefer a more textured soup, purée half and add it to the non-puréed half. Stir well.

Pour the oil into a large stockpot or saucepan, and add the celeriac, celery, onions and sweet pepper. Cover the pan and set it over a medium heat. Sauté the vegetables for 20 minutes, stirring occasionally.

When the vegetables are very tender, add the paprika and stir well.

Add the stock, then use a hand-held blender to purée the soup. Stir in the chestnut purée and bring the soup to a low simmer.

Remove from the heat and serve immediately or chill in the refrigerator for reheating and serving the next day.

✱ **CELERIAC (CELERY ROOT)** looks a most unlikely object to be edible. It is brown, lumpy, rough-textured and, unless the grocer has got to it first, arrives with various rampant tentacle-like appendages growing out of each knobbly bit. But pare away the mucky armour plating and you have a food to celebrate. When cooked it is tender, with a lovely cream-coloured flesh beneath its gnarled skin, and a subtle flavour of celery. Rinse it and chop, grate, steam or stir-fry it; you can even eat it raw. It keeps well in the salad drawer of the refrigerator and cooks quickly.

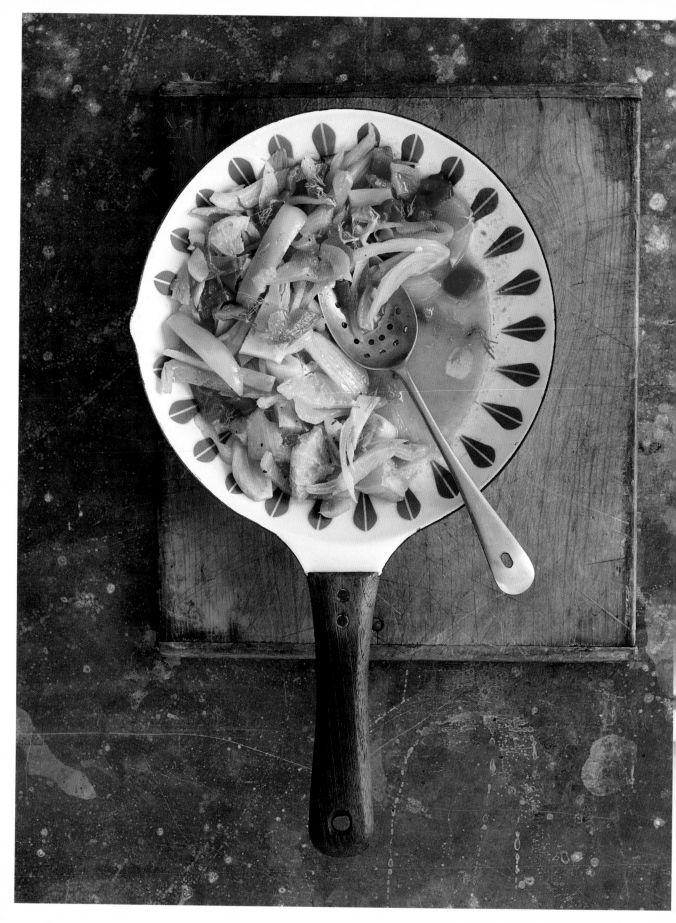

FENNEL AND PEPPER PRESTO

There are times when a salad appeals – except that you really want something warm. This fits the bill perfectly. It will actually take you longer to prepare the ingredients than it will to cook this dish. For interest, use different coloured peppers (one green, the other yellow perhaps) and create texture by being creative with the way you cut the ingredients. Serve as a side dish to Tofu and Couscous Magic (page 126), Tempeh Crisps in Pomegranate Glaze (page 167) or Three-Grain Risotto (page 184).

SERVES 4

PREPARATION TIME 20 MINUTES

1 large orange, peeled and divided into four sections

1 tablespoon untoasted sesame oil

1 fennel (finocchio) bulb, very thinly sliced

1 small sweet pepper (capsicum), deseeded and sliced into quarter rounds or long strips

1 hot fresh chilli, deseeded and thinly sliced

4 spring onions (scallions), cut into chunks

12 garlic cloves, sliced

1 medium tomato, chopped

Salt and pepper, to taste

OPTIONS AND VARIATIONS

Add ¼ teaspoon crushed fennel seeds or a few feathery fronds of fresh fennel in the last minute of cooking.

Prepare all the ingredients first, and have them ready in separate bowls for when you start cooking.

Slice the orange quarters across the segments to create little fan shapes. Slicing will release some juice, which you should try to retain.

Pour the oil into a large frying pan (skillet) set over a high heat. When the oil is hot, add the fennel, pepper, chilli, spring onions and garlic, and cover the pan for 2 minutes. Stir the ingredients and cover the pan again for 2 minutes.

Add the tomato and orange slices, and stir well. Cover the pan, and let the fennel mixture cook for 1 minute. Turn off the heat, but leave the pan on the stove for 1 minute.

Turn the vegetables into a serving dish, pouring over any orange juice you managed to retain. Season with salt and pepper, and serve.

LEEK AND POTATO SOUP

I used to think I could actually see our sons growing as they ate this soup. It is thick and nutritious with an appealing aroma. The flavour deepens if you make it ahead of time: pop the whole pot in the refrigerator and serve the soup the next day. It is reviving and sustaining, especially if served with a thick chunk of Seeded Spelt Bread (page 87).

SERVES 4

PREPARATION TIME 40 MINUTES

1 tablespoon untoasted sesame oil

3 medium potatoes, roughly diced

2 large leeks, cleaned and trimmed as described in note

2 large onions, chopped

1 teaspoon caraway seeds

1 teaspoon vegan bouillon powder

½ teaspoon black pepper

1 litre (35fl oz/4 cups) vegetable stock or water

2 sprigs of fresh parsley, leaves picked and finely chopped

1 small carrot, grated

OPTIONS AND VARIATIONS

Sometimes, if the leeks don't have quite enough green left on their stalk, the soup can look too pale. In this case, stir a scant ¼ teaspoon ground turmeric into the saucepan, before bringing it to the simmer.

Pour the oil into a large stockpot or saucepan, and layer these ingredients in the pan in the following order: potatoes, leeks, onions, caraway seeds, bouillon powder and then the pepper. Cover the pan and set it over a medium heat. Stir the contents after about 10 minutes, then cover and cook for a further 10–12 minutes until the vegetables are tender.

Add the stock, and stir well. Purée the soup to the consistency you prefer using a hand-held blender.

Add the parsley and carrot, and bring the soup to a low simmer. Remove from the heat and, if you're not eating immediately, leave the pan covered until you're ready to serve.

✱ **CLEANING LEEKS** I always try to use as much of a leek as possible: the green section is very nutritious and tasty, and should not be wasted. As leeks grow, their growers mound up the soil around them to stop the whole stalk from turning green. This practice results in the long, tender white section, which is so distinctive. However, there can be a lot of soil hiding in the upper parts of the leek as a result, so you need to clean them carefully. I start by washing the whole leek and trimming away the root and any ragged tips of the leaves. I discard any yellowed or very fibrous outer layers, then slice the leek into rings. I put the rings into a bowl of cold water. Rather than tipping them into a colander to drain them, I use my hands to lift the leek rings out of the water so that any soil is left behind. I rinse them under cold running water, and then they are ready to use.

CREAM OF MUSHROOM SOUP

Fresh mushrooms bring the flavour of autumn (fall) into your kitchen. The supermarkets provide common types all the year round, but the seasonal mushroom stall at your local farmers' market can offer greater variety and interest. A slice of Seeded Spelt Bread (page 87) dipped in a little extra virgin olive oil is all you need to go with this.

SERVES 4

PREPARATION TIME 1 HOUR

2 tablespoons untoasted sesame oil

200g (7oz) mushrooms, finely chopped

1 large onion, finely chopped

1 whole garlic bulb, cloves separated and chopped

4 tablespoons plain (all-purpose) or wholemeal (whole-wheat) flour

1 teaspoon vegan bouillon powder

½ teaspoon ground turmeric

½ teaspoon Chinese five-spice

¼ teaspoon black pepper

1 litre (35fl oz/4 cups) unsweetened soya milk

500ml (17fl ox/2 cups) vegetable stock or water

Pour the oil into a large stockpot or saucepan set over a low to medium heat. Add the mushroom, onion and garlic, and sauté for 15 minutes, covering the pan but stirring occasionally. The mushrooms should be well cooked; the onions and garlic very tender.

Mix together the flour, bouillon, turmeric, Chinese five-spice and pepper in a bowl. In a measuring jug (large measuring cup), combine half of the soya milk with the stock.

When the mushrooms are ready, sprinkle over the dry mixture and stir constantly as the mixture thickens, for about 3 minutes.

Keep stirring the mushroom mixture as you pour the liquid mixture into the pan, about 100ml (3½fl oz/½ cup) at a time. Allow each addition of liquid to be incorporated before adding the next. When the whole amount has been added, let the soup cook for 15 minutes, covered, over a low heat.

Adjust the consistency of the soup if you wish by adding more soya milk, a little at a time, stirring frequently. When you are happy with the consistency, let the soup warm to nearly simmering and serve.

SAUTÉED TATSOI WITH BLACK SESAME

Only three ingredients and a little seasoning make this dish simple and quick to prepare. The partnership of juicy greens and nutty black sesame is irresistible. Wonderful served with Onion and Potato Flip (page 46) or Carrot, Arame and Ginger Sauté (page 195).

SERVES 4

PREPARATION TIME 15 MINUTES

400–600g (14–20oz) fresh tatsoi or pak choi (bok choy)

½–1 tablespoon untoasted sesame oil

2 tablespoons black sesame seeds

Salt and pepper, to taste

OPTIONS AND VARIATIONS

Add 4 garlic cloves, sliced, when adding the tatsoi. Add 1 small tomato, chopped, when you turn the tatsoi. Use pak choi (bok choy) if tatsoi is not available.

Trim the root end of the tatsoi, cutting through about 4cm (1¾in) from the base of the bunch, so that the stalks (with their attached leaves) separate.

Heat a large frying pan (skillet) over a medium heat and add ½ tablespoon of the sesame oil. Swirl it around the pan, then add the sesame seeds and spread them around the pan.

Add the tatsoi to the pan, keeping the stems all pointing in one direction. Cover the pan and leave to cook for 5 minutes. Use a spatula or kitchen tongs to turn the tatsoi. The tatsoi should release a lot of its juices, in which case you will not need to add any more oil. If the tatsoi is not very fresh, or is at the end of its season, it may not release much moisture. If this is the case, add a little more of the sesame oil to the pan.

Cover the pan and cook a further 5 minutes until the tatsoi leaves are wilted and the stems tender but retaining some crispness. Just before serving, turn the tatsoi to coat it nicely with the sesame seeds. Season the greens with salt and pepper, and serve hot.

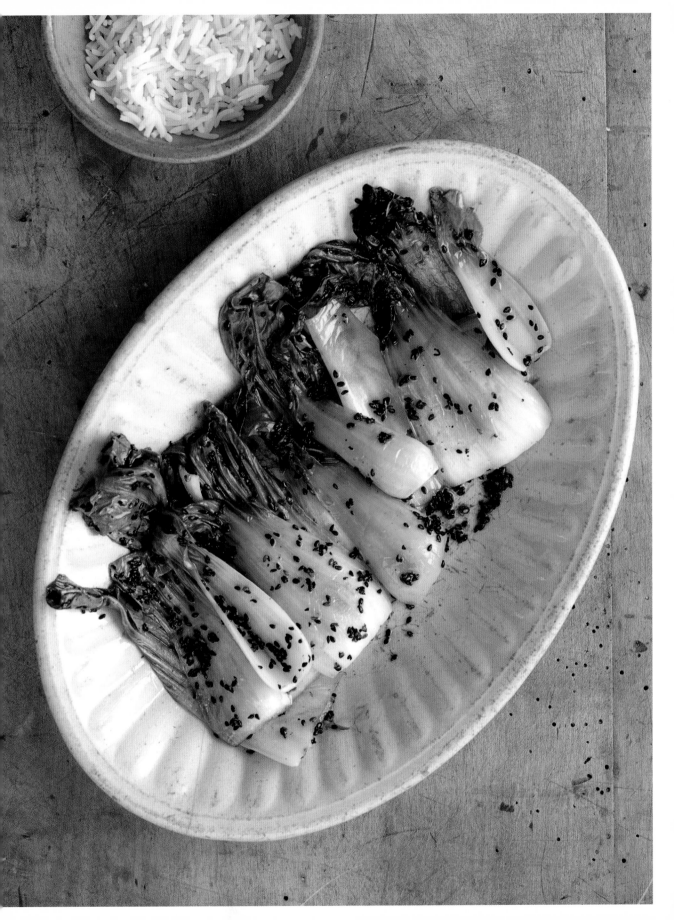

STIR-FRIED VEGETABLES WITH SPICED NOODLES

Adjust the ingredients in your stir-fry to suit the season. Have everything prepared before you start to cook – it all happens rather quickly! Top with roasted cashews, marinated tofu and a sprinkle of tamari.

SERVES 4

PREPARATION TIME 40 MINUTES

½ teaspoon Chinese five-spice

¼ teaspoon cayenne pepper

10cm (4in) strip of kombu, rinsed

2 tablespoons untoasted sesame oil

200g (7oz) dried noodles

BOWL 1

2 celery stalks, sliced

2 medium carrots, thinly sliced into 5–8cm (2–3in) lengths

BOWL 2

12 baby sweetcorn, halved lengthways

½ head of broccoli, florets cut into quarters

125g (4½oz) French (string) beans, trimmed and sliced in half (about 1 cup prepared)

BOWL 3

1 medium courgette (zucchini), cut into coins

200g (7oz) tatsoi or pak choi (bok choy)

2 tablespoons grated fresh ginger

1 fresh chilli, thinly sliced

6 garlic cloves, sliced

3 spring onions (scallions), chopped

In preparation for cooking the noodles, fill a large pan with water. Add the five-spice powder, cayenne and kombu, cover the pan and set over a medium heat to come to the boil.

Set a wok or large pan over a medium heat. When it is hot, add the oil. Immediately add the contents of bowl 1 to the pan. Stir once, cover the pan, and cook for about 5 minutes.

Add the contents of bowl 2 to the pan. Stir well and cover for about 5 minutes.

The water for the noodles should be boiling now. Add the noodles to the water, and cook for according to the packet instructions (usually about 8 minutes) while you finish stir-frying the vegetables. Use kitchen tongs to separate the noodles as they cook.

Meanwhile, add the contents of bowl 3 to the stir-fry. Stir well and cover the pan. Cook for about 3 minutes, then remove from the heat and leave the pan covered.

When the noodles are ready, drain them and divide them among four plates or bowls. Spoon the vegetable stir-fry over the noodles and serve.

SPICY CAULIFLOWER IN CREAMY ONION SAUCE

The cauliflower is quick to cook, but give this sauce time to cook slowly. The onions must gently soften without browning, so that the sauce remains creamy in both colour and texture. The flavour is delicate but distinctive. Draw a pattern with this sauce on the surface of a bowl of Ruby Root Soup (page 248), or serve as a hot dipping sauce with Polenta with Garden Garland (page 100).

SERVES 4

PREPARATION TIME 45 MINUTES

2 large white-fleshed onions, finely chopped

250ml (9fl oz/1 cup) vegetable stock or water

1 tablespoon untoasted sesame oil

1 tablespoon plain (all-purpose) flour

250ml (9fl oz/1 cup) coconut milk

1 tablespoon coconut oil

1 head of cauliflower, florets halved

1 fresh chilli, finely chopped

1 medium tomato, chopped

Salt, to taste

OPTIONS AND VARIATIONS

Add ¼ teaspoon of ground nutmeg when stirring in the flour.

Start with the sauce. Put the chopped onions and one-quarter of the cauliflower florets in a saucepan with the stock, and set over a medium heat. Cover the pan and simmer until very tender, about 15 minutes.

Strain the cooking liquid into a measuring jug (large measuring cup) and set to one side. Transfer the cooked onion and cauliflower to a bowl and mash (or pass through a Mouli); set aside.

Pour the sesame oil into the saucepan and set over a medium heat. Sprinkle the flour over the hot oil and stir to create a thick paste.

Add the coconut milk to the reserved cooking liquid in the jug and stir well. Gradually add this liquid to the paste in the pan, stirring after each addition, to create a smooth, thick sauce.

Stir in the mashed onions and cauliflower, add a pinch of salt and cook for a further 2–3 minutes. Cover the pan and remove from the heat.

For the spicy cauliflower, place a frying pan over a high heat. Add the coconut oil, then add the rest of the cauliflower and the chilli. Cover the pan and cook for 3–5 minutes, then turn the ingredients and add the tomato. Cover and cook a further 3–5 minutes. Turn into a serving dish and dress with the Creamy Onion Sauce. Serve.

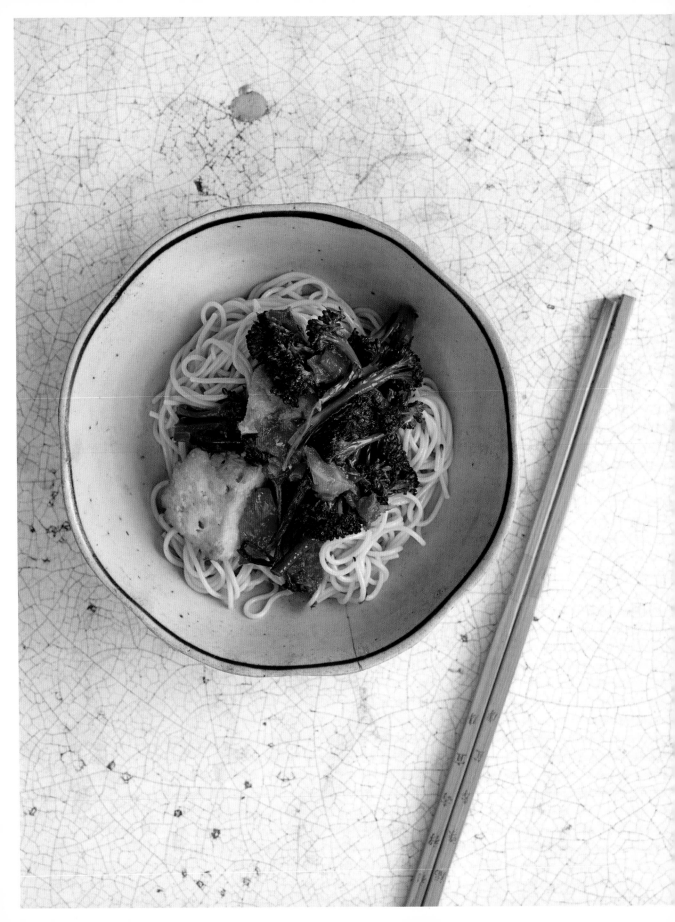

CHUNKY TOFU IN GREENS

It's easy to tailor this dish to suit the season and the type of greens available. Try leaf greens such as pak choi (bok choy), chopped watercress or curly kale instead of the broccoli. The chunkiness of the tofu appeals to omnivores and vegans alike. Use this stir-fry as filling for a baked potato or with Yellow Rice Zinger (page 129). It is also excellent served over noodles, with a topping of Hot Peanut Sauce (page 246).

Put the tofu chunks in a large pan with the oil; cover and place over a high heat for 3 minutes. Reduce the heat and use a spatula to turn the tofu chunks. Aim to keep the chunks intact with a little bit of browning or crisping on each side.

After about 15 minutes, add the garlic and broccoli, using the spatula to stir the ingredients. Cover the pan and cook for about 5 minutes. Use the spatula to turn the ingredients again.

Add the tomatoes and oregano, cover the pan and cook for a further 5 minutes until the broccoli is just tender but still bright green. Season with salt and pepper, and serve.

SERVES 4

PREPARATION TIME 45 MINUTES

400g (14oz) firm tofu, cubed (about 2¼ cups prepared)

2 tablespoons untoasted sesame oil

1 whole garlic bulb, cloves separated and chopped

1 head of broccoli, florets halved or quartered

2 medium tomatoes, chopped

½ teaspoon dried oregano

Salt and pepper, to taste

OPTIONS AND VARIATIONS

If you prefer a spicy dish, add 1 thinly sliced fresh chilli. Use 12–15 Brussels sprouts, halved, instead of the broccoli. Add 4 chopped spring onions (scallions).

FOUR-DAY SOURDOUGH BREAD

If you value patience, making this bread this will prove you have it. Sourdough cannot be rushed, but it can inspire you to reconnect with the long tradition of bread-making using naturally occurring 'wild' yeast cultures.

MAKES 2 LOAVES

PREPARATION TIME 4 DAYS

FOR THE STARTER

225g (8oz/2½ cups) plain (all-purpose) or wholemeal (whole-wheat) flour, plus 4 tablespoons more for 'feeding'

FOR THE BREAD

1kg (2¼lb) plain (all-purpose) or wholemeal (whole-wheat) flour

3 tablespoons extra virgin olive oil, plus a little extra for greasing the pans

To make the starter, put the flour and 300ml (10½fl oz/1¼ cups) water into a wide-necked jar and mix well. Cover the neck of the jar with a piece of muslin (cheesecloth) held in place by a rubber band. Leave to stand in a warm, draught-free place for 24 hours.

Add 2 tablespoons flour and 3 tablespoons water to the jar and mix well. Cover the jar and leave in a warm place for another 24 hours.

Repeat this process once more on the third day.

On the fourth day, you should see a few small bubbles on the surface of the starter. Check that it smells nice (you will know if it doesn't) and whisk it again. You're now ready to make the bread!

Put the flour in a large bowl and measure 400ml (14fl oz) warm water into a jug (large measuring cup). Stir the starter and add at least 300ml (10½fl oz/1¼ cups) of it to the flour. Add the 3 tablespoons olive oil and stir with a wooden spoon until it becomes difficult. Begin to knead the dough with your hands, adding some of the warm water, little by little, to create a firm dough that is not sticky.

Knead the dough for 5 minutes. Cover the bowl with a cloth and leave the dough to rise for 2–4 hours.

Lightly oil two 900g (2lb) loaf pans. Knead the dough again and divide into two. Shape into loaves and place in the prepared pans. Cover the loaves and leave to rise for 2 hours.

Preheat the oven to 200°C (400°F). Bake the loaves at this temperature for 5 minutes, then reduce the oven temperature to 180°C (350°C) and bake for a further 25 minutes. Leave to cool in the pans for 5 minutes, then turn out onto a wire rack.

✳ **TO KEEP YOUR STARTER GOING** After you've used some of the starter to leaven a dough, you can replenish it by feeding it, ready for the next time you want to make bread. To 'feed' it, add more flour and water in approximately these proportions: 1 part flour (of any sort or a mixture) to 1¼ parts water. As long as you replenish it in this way, the starter will remain viable. Use as much as you need for your next batch of bread (about 300ml/10½fl oz/1¼ cups), but keep a small amount to inoculate the next batch of starter. If you plan to use the starter quite soon, keep it at an ambient temperature and feed it every day. If you want to keep it for a longer period, store in the refrigerator and feed it twice a week.

STEAMED SWEET POTATO WITH GINGER AND NORI DRESSING

The sweet potato has such a special flavour, so it is easy to cook it simply. Here, I add the intense flavours of this highly versatile dressing. It's one of my favourites, which I often use to dress steamed vegetables served with a portion of ramen or soba noodles. I also use it as a dipping sauce or marinade, or on baked potatoes or bean sprouts. Spoon a little onto a burger made from Quick Patty Cake Mix (page 50) or marinate a few pieces of fried tempeh or tofu for the next day. The dressing benefits from sitting for a while before use.

To make the dressing, stir together the ginger, lemon juice, olive oil, vinegar, tamari and nori flakes in a small bowl. Cover and leave to stand for at least 2 hours if possible, to allow the flavours to blend.

Place the sweet potato chips in a steaming basket over 3cm (1¼in) of water. Cover and bring to the boil, then steam for 7–10 minutes. These are delicious as they are, but, if you want to caramelize them a little, transfer the steamed chips to a tray or baking sheet with the untoasted sesame oil. Toss to cover and place under a preheated hot grill (broiler) for 5 minutes.

Serve the chips with a small dipping pot of the dressing, or drizzle a spoonful of the dressing over each portion.

SERVES 4

PREPARATION TIME 30 MINUTES

+ 2 HOURS STANDING

2 tablespoons grated fresh ginger

Juice of 1 lemon

4 tablespoons extra virgin olive oil

2 tablespoons apple cider vinegar

1 tablespoon tamari

1 tablespoon nori flakes

450g (1lb) sweet potato, cut into thick chips (fries)

1 tablespoon untoasted sesame oil

OPTIONS AND VARIATIONS

Add 1 crushed garlic clove.

✳ **STEAMING VEGETABLES** Say 'steamed vegetables' and it sounds as if you are describing a queue of grumpy, road-weary veg standing by the extractor fan outside a dry cleaners. Not so! Steaming helps fresh vegetables to retain more nutrients, more flavour and more texture than if you were to boil them. It is remarkably quick and also saves energy because you can stack food in layers above one pot of boiling water. I use both types: a basket steamer, which concertinas in size to fit inside most pans, and a stacking steamer. I can do three layers in a stack, and I can add and remove layers, too, as they finish cooking. Steamed vegetables don't need a recipe. Sometimes they need a little sauce or dressing, but they are so naturally flavoursome that I recommend a light touch, especially while you get to know them.

SPLENDID WHOLESOME LOAF

Fill your home with the enticing aroma of baking bread by making a batch of these stalwart loaves. I always bake four at a time and, more often than not, one of them is sampled and gone within a few hours! Though a treat when still warm, this bread slices better after it has cooled. It freezes well and a loaf wrapped in baking paper is a lovely gift to give a friend. I serve toasted slices of this under Stalybridge Beans-on-Toast (page 52) or Scrambled Tofu (page 39), or dip it into bowlfuls of Alphabet Soup (page 95) or Garden Nettle Soup (page 74).

MAKES 4 LOAVES

PREPARATION TIME 3 HOURS

2 teaspoons sugar

1 × 8g sachet or 2 teaspoons dried yeast

1.5kg (3lb 5oz) wholemeal (whole-wheat) flour

500g (1lb 2oz) wholemeal (wholegrain) spelt flour

2 tablespoons extra virgin olive oil, plus extra for oiling the pans

OPTIONS AND VARIATIONS

You can adjust the proportions of the two flours in this recipe, if you happen to have more of one than the other. Try reversing the proportions: use 1.5kg (3lb 5oz) spelt and 500g (1lb 2oz) wholemeal (whole-wheat) flour. Or use strong white bread flour instead of the spelt flour if that's what you have in the cupboard.

Measure 500ml (17fl oz/2 cups) warm water into a measuring jug (large measuring cup) and dissolve the sugar in it. Add the yeast, stir well and set the mixture aside to turn frothy.

Mix the flours together in a large bowl.

When the yeast is frothy, stir in the oil and then pour the yeast and oil mixture into the flour. Begin to stir with a wooden spoon, adding another 500ml (17fl oz/2 cups) warm water as you stir.

When stirring becomes difficult, knead the dough by hand for at least 5 minutes until it has a firm but slightly moist consistency. Aim to knead in all of the flour – it can be hard work – adding more warm water if needed, but in very small amounts to prevent the dough becoming too soft and sticky.

Eventually, very little or none of the dough should stick to your hands. You'll notice the dough becoming more elastic. This will give the loaf a light texture.

Shape the dough into a ball in the bowl and cover the bowl with a clean cloth. Set aside in a warm place for about 1 hour to allow the dough to rise – you want it to roughly double in size.

Meanwhile, lightly oil four 900g (2lb) loaf pans.

When the dough has risen, put a little oil on your hands and knead the dough for 2–3 minutes. Divide the dough into four parts, shape the portions into loaves and place each one in an oiled pan. Cover the pans with a cloth and leave to rise for another hour.

Preheat the oven to 250°C (500°F). Arrange the pans in the hot oven so they are not too close together. Bake for 5 minutes, then reduce the oven temperature to 180°C (350°F) and bake for a further 25 minutes until the loaves are browned on top and give a hollow sound when tapped on the bottom.

Turn out the loaves onto a wire rack and leave to cool.

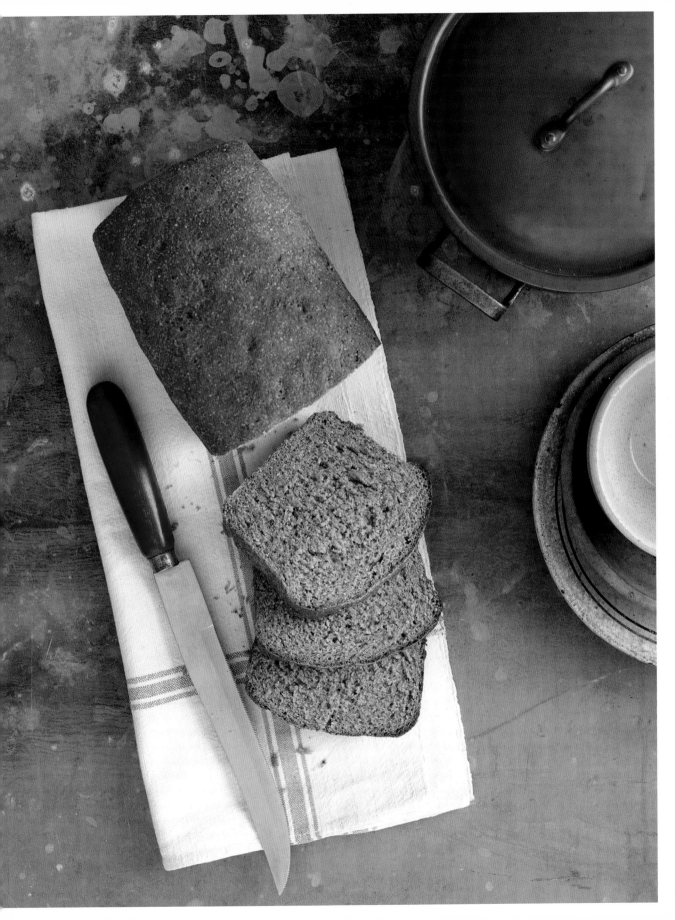

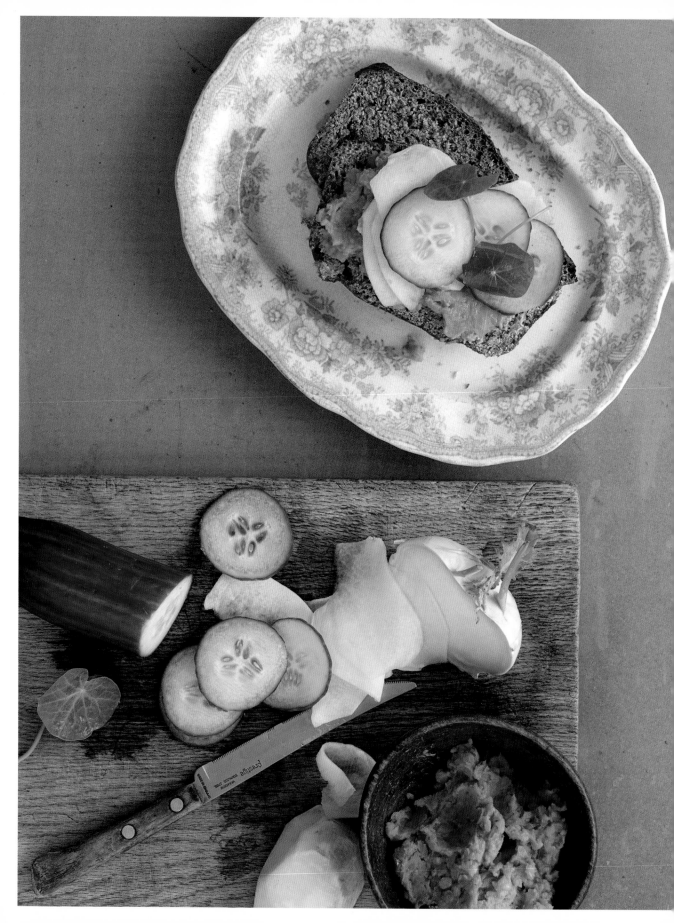

SPEEDY SANDWICH COLLECTION

Here are four sandwiches that move off the plate very quickly. Fortunately, they are almost as quick to make!

KOHLRABI AND CUCUMBER SANDWICH A slightly crisp, refreshing snack. Spread slices of fresh or toasted bread with Herb and Onion Bean Butter (page 71). Arrange layers of thinly sliced kohlrabi and thinly sliced cucumber on one slice of bread, seasoning each layer with salt and pepper as you go. If you like, you can spread a little Tofu-Mayo (page 99) between the layers. For a peppery taste, add finely chopped nasturtium leaves. Top with another slice of bread.

AVOCADO ROCKET LAUNCH SANDWICH Scoop the flesh of 1 ripe avocado into a bowl and add 1 finely chopped ripe tomato and about 25g (1oz/½ cup) chopped fresh rocket (arugula). Mix well, using a fork to mash the avocado and press the juices from the tomato. Spread the mixture onto 4 slices of fresh or toasted bread, season with salt and pepper, and sandwich the slices together in pairs. If you like, you can use toasted pitta instead of sliced bread, or sprinkle Sprouted Mung Beans (page 78) over the filling before closing the sandwiches.

MISO AND TAHINI PROTEIN-BOOSTER SANDWICH Mix together 4 tablespoons tahini and 1 tablespoon miso in a bowl, to create a thick paste. Spread the paste on 2 slices of hot toasted bread, and sandwich them together. Optional extras include adding a dash of Tabasco or hot sauce before you close the sandwich, or stirring the juice of ½ lemon into the tahini and miso paste.

BANANA AND PEANUT BUTTER CLASSIC PLUS Spread 4 tablespoons peanut butter onto 2 slices of fresh or toasted bread. Slice 1 ripe banana and layer over the peanut butter. Sprinkle a pinch of ground cinnamon over the banana slices, grate over a little plain dark chocolate, and serve. For extra sweetness, drizzle 1 teaspoon of barley malt syrup over the creation before you close the sandwich. Try using tahini instead of peanut butter, for a flavour akin to the Middle Eastern confection halva.

EASY PIZZA BASE

Here's a light, slightly crisp base for your pizza. Top with a little Rich Tomato Sauce (page 253) and experiment with toppings such as thinly sliced tomatoes with finely cubed basil tofu or some Tempeh Crisps (page 167). Alternatively, try Simple Herb and Caper Pizza (page 125) or Extremely Olive Pizza (page 236).

MAKES 2 × 30cm (12in) BASES

PREPARATION TIME 1 HOUR

1 heaped teaspoon sugar

1 × 8g sachet or 2 teaspoons dried yeast

500g (1lb 2oz/4 cups) strong white bread flour

2 tablespoons extra virgin olive oil

Measure 250ml (9fl oz/1 cup) warm (blood temperature) water into a measuring jug (large measuring cup), and dissolve the sugar in it. Add the yeast, stir well and set the mixture aside to turn frothy.

Measure the flour into a large bowl and make a well in the centre. Add 1 tablespoon of the oil to the jug containing the yeast mixture. Stir gently and pour the whole lot into the flour.

Measure another 100ml (3½fl oz/scant ½ cup) warm water into the jug and keep it handy.

Stir the flour and liquid together with a wooden spoon until it becomes difficult. Scrape the dough off the spoon and begin to knead the dough with your hand, adding a little of the extra 100ml (3½fl oz/scant ½ cup) water if needed. Aim to make a dough that is firm but slightly sticky.

Cover the bowl with a towel, and leave the dough to rise for 20 minutes.

Use the remaining oil to lightly grease two 30cm (12in) pizza trays or sheets. Use your hands to distribute the oil – the oil will stop the dough sticking to your hands when you handle the dough in the next step.

Divide the dough in two and gently press each portion, gradually spreading it to the edges of the pizza tray.

Set the trays aside to let the dough rise for 20–30 minutes while you prepare the toppings of your choice.

❋ **MAKING DOUGH** All flours can be temperamental: they will absorb liquids to a different extent each day depending on the weather, the temperature and how recently they were ground into flour. We have to work with this. When making a dough, it's a good idea to have a little extra water ready (as described above), just in case you need it. That way you don't drag bits of ragged, floury dough all over the place while you try to refill the measuring jug. But it is wise to add liquids a little at a time, so that you don't make your dough too wet. That would require you to add more flour, then more water ... and so on!

SIMPLE HERB AND CAPER PIZZA

You and your family can form the delivery service for this light but flavoursome treat. I keep the necessary ingredients in the cupboard for emergency pizza requests and, with everyone doing one part of the prep, it arrives on the table very fast. Excellent with Quickly Salad (page 93) and Avocado Almond Shake (page 68).

MAKES 2 × 30cm (12in) PIZZAS

PREPARATION TIME 1 HOUR

1 quantity Easy Pizza Base (opposite)

2 teaspoons untoasted sesame oil

1 whole garlic bulb, cloves separated and finely chopped

½ teaspoon chilli flakes

1 tablespoon dried basil

1 teaspoon dried oregano

100g (3½oz/about ¾ cup) sun-dried tomatoes, finely chopped

500g (1lb 2oz) passata (tomato purée)

100g (3½oz) capers, rinsed and dried

OPTIONS AND VARIATIONS

Use Your Own Tomato Compote (page 254) instead of the passata listed here. Grate 150g (5½oz) vegan Cheddar-type cheese, and sprinkle half onto each pizza during the last 5 minutes of baking.

Prepare the pizza base recipe first and, while the dough is rising in the trays, make the sauce.

Measure the oil into a saucepan, and sauté the garlic and chilli flakes over a medium heat. When the garlic is tender, after about 5 minutes, add the herbs and sun-dried tomatoes. Cook for 2–3 minutes until the mixture is softened and aromatic. Add the passata, stir well and bring to a low simmer.

Preheat the oven to 200°C (400°F).

When the dough is ready, ladle half of the sauce onto each base, spreading it almost to the edge. Evenly scatter half the capers over each pizza.

Bake in the oven for 5 minutes (to ensure a crisp base), before reducing the temperature to 180°C (350°F) and baking for a further 15 minutes until the edges of the dough are golden brown.

Remove the pizzas from the oven. Slice and serve immediately.

TOFU AND COUSCOUS MAGIC

I count this as one of the twelve dishes that young adults can learn to cook before they leave home. It's quick, versatile, healthy and stimulates an interest in cooking creatively. Serve on its own for a warming and sustaining one-bowl meal, with tamari, sriracha sauce or the juice of a lime. For added texture, try sprinkling a handful of Roasted Seed Mixture (page 86) over your portion.

SERVES 4

PREPARATION TIME 25 MINUTES

1 tablespoon untoasted sesame oil

1 medium onion, finely chopped

4 garlic cloves, chopped

1 teaspoon dried basil or mixed dried herbs

¼ teaspoon black pepper

400g (14oz) firm tofu, cut into small cubes (about 2¼ cups)

200g (7oz) tatsoi or pak choi (bok choy), sliced

250g (9oz/1⅓ cups) medium couscous

OPTIONS AND VARIATIONS

You can use any greens that appeal, if they will cook in the time you have available. One surprise version of this dish successfully included a mixture of chopped cos (romaine) lettuce, fresh flat-leaf parsley and fresh basil. Fresh or dried chilli may be used instead of the black pepper.

Put the oil in a large saucepan, and sauté the onion and garlic over a medium heat for 5 minutes. Add the basil, pepper, tofu and greens. Stir well and cover the pan. Continue cooking for 10 minutes until the greens are tender.

Add the dry couscous and stir well. Pour in 400ml (14fl oz) water, stir well and cover the pan. The couscous will absorb the juices and water very quickly. After 2–3 minutes, check the texture of the couscous. It should not be granular, but instead tender and fluffy. If necessary, add a little more water, stir and cover the pan. Check the texture again after 2–3 minutes.

When the couscous is ready, turn off the heat and leave to stand for 5 minutes before serving.

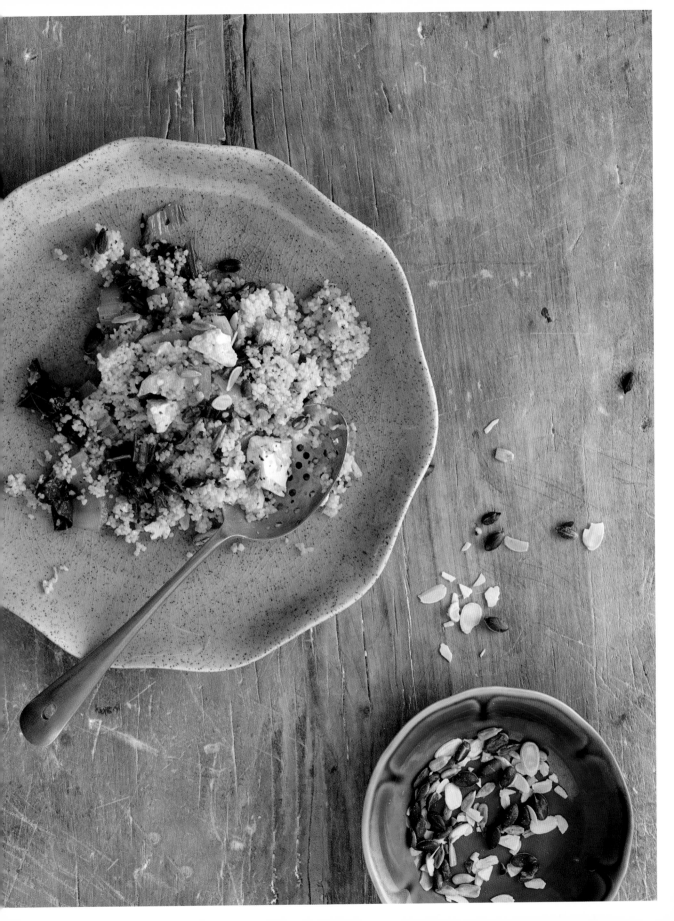

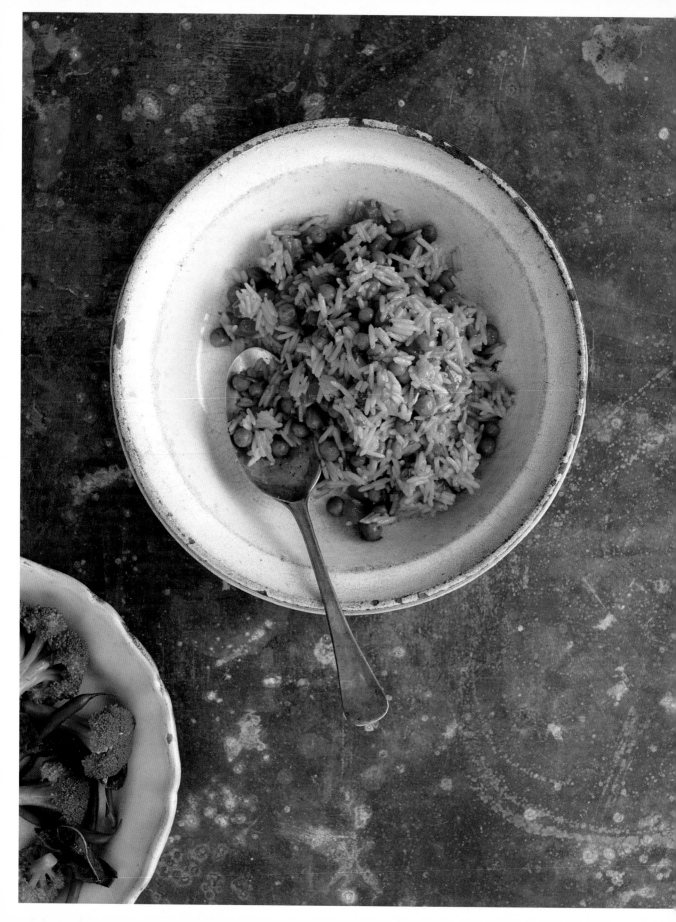

YELLOW RICE ZINGER

This pretty dish is spicy, colourful and versatile. It's excellent served hot with sides of beans or greens, or cold alongside a salad. Thanks to the spices and basmati rice, it is highly aromatic. Try it with Dressed Greens and Beans (page 154) or Adzuki Bean Ragout (page 134).

(page 154) ... (page 134)

SERVES 4

PREPARATION TIME 30 MINUTES

2 tablespoons untoasted sesame oil

1 whole garlic bulb, cloves separated and chopped

1 sweet red pepper (capsicum), diced

1 teaspoon vegan bouillon powder

½ teaspoon ground turmeric

½ teaspoon chilli flakes

¼ teaspoon ground cinnamon

¼ teaspoon cumin seeds

250g (9oz/1¼ cups) basmati rice

25g (1oz/½ cup) chopped fresh flat-leaf parsley

250g (9oz/1⅔ cups) fresh or frozen green peas

OPTIONS AND VARIATIONS

Add 50g (1¾oz/½ cup) flaked almonds or pine nuts when you add the parsley and peas. Add 2 tablespoons chopped fresh basil just before serving.

Measure the oil into a large saucepan; sauté the garlic and sweet pepper over a medium heat for about 5 minutes. Add the bouillon powder and spices. Stir well and cook a further 2 minutes.

Stir in the basmati and keep stirring while it absorbs the oil and the flavours of the cooked mixture. Add 500ml (17fl oz/2 cups) water, stir well and cover the pan.

After about 5 minutes, add the parsley and peas, stirring well. Cover the pan and allow time for the liquid to be absorbed, another 5–7 minutes. Your aim is to have rice that is tender and fluffy but not wet, and for the peas and parsley to cook but remain fairly bright. If necessary, add more water in small amounts, up to 100ml (3½fl oz/ scant ½ cup), and continue cooking until it is absorbed.

When everything is cooked, remove the pan from the heat. Fluff the rice as you serve it.

MEDITERRANEAN SPICED RICE AND LENTILS

I can never seem to make enough of this versatile dish. It's good served hot or cold, with salads or hot vegetables, and it transports well for a packed lunch or picnic. This recipe makes a generous quantity – enough to keep a tub of it on standby in the refrigerator for snacks or late breakfasts. It is unavoidably brown, but it lights up when served with something more colourful. I think it looks very appealing served hot alongside Carrot, Arame and Ginger Sauté (page 195) and Precious Greens (page 193), or served cold beside Entirely Green Salad (page 92) and a plate of sliced tomatoes.

SERVES 4

PREPARATION TIME 45 MINUTES

250g (9oz/1¼ cups) brown lentils, rinsed

3 tablespoons untoasted sesame oil

1 large onion, finely chopped

1 whole garlic bulb, cloves separated and finely chopped

1 teaspoon chilli flakes

1 teaspoon cumin seeds

½ teaspoon ground cinnamon

250g (9oz1¼ cups) basmati rice

4 spring onions (scallions), finely chopped

OPTIONS AND VARIATIONS

Add 1 teaspoon vegan bouillon powder when you add the spices.

Tip the lentils into a saucepan and cover with boiling water. Cover the pan and leave to stand for 15–20 minutes

Meanwhile, pour the oil into a large saucepan set over a medium heat. Add the onion and garlic, and sauté for 5 minutes, stirring often. Add the spices, stir well and reduce the heat. Sauté for a further 5 minutes.

Now add the rice and stir well. Leave it to cook for 5 minutes, stirring once or twice to help the rice absorb the spice flavours.

Drain and rinse the soaked lentils, then add them to the pan, stirring them into the rice and spice mixture. Increase the heat to medium, and cover the rice and lentil mixture with boiling water to a depth of 1.5cm (⅝in). Stir well, cover the pan and leave to cook for 10–12 minutes.

Stir the spring onions into the mixture and check the consistency. Aim for both rice and lentils to be hydrated and tender, but not wet – if needed, add a little more boiling water to the pan and keep it over the heat for another 5 minutes.

When the rice and lentils are cooked, remove the cover from the pan to allow some of the steam to evaporate. Serve hot or cold.

ONION, TOFU AND TOMATO TART

Rocket (arugula) is not usually thought of as a green you'd cook, but it has a peppery 'bite' that adds depth to this dish. I find that tofu can sometimes 'mute' the flavours of other ingredients, so go ahead and adjust the amount of spice to suit your own tastes. This tart is excellent with Entirely Green Salad (page 92), Sautéed Tatsoi with Black Sesame (page 112) or Carrot, Arame and Ginger Sauté (page 195).

MAKES 1 × 28cm (11in) TART

PREPARATION TIME 1 HOUR

½ quantity Vegan Shortcrust Pastry (page 265)

1 large carrot, thinly sliced

25g (1oz/¾ cup) chopped fresh flat-leaf parsley

2 large onions, finely chopped

50g (1¾oz/1½ cups) fresh rocket (arugula), finely chopped

2 medium tomatoes, thinly sliced

250g (9oz) plain firm tofu, cubed (about 1⅓ cups prepared)

150ml (5fl oz) soya milk

1 teaspoon black pepper

1 teaspoon dried basil

½ teaspoon dried oregano

½ teaspoon ground turmeric

OPTIONS AND VARIATIONS

Use watercress in place of the rocket. Add 2 tablespoons nutritional yeast flakes, or 2 tablespoons prepared mustard, to the tofu and milk mixture.

Take the prepared pastry out of the refrigerator about 30 minutes before you need it.

Preheat the oven to 180°C (350°F) and line a 28cm (11¼in) pie dish with the pastry. Arrange the carrot slices over the pastry, ensuring that they are placed right to the edges of the pastry base. Scatter the parsley evenly over the carrot slices and the onions over the parsley. Distribute the rocket over the onion and arrange the tomato slices on top of the rocket.

In a bowl, purée the tofu, soya milk, pepper, herbs and turmeric using a hand-held blender. Pour the tofu mixture over the tart, ensuring even distribution.

Bake in the oven for 30–35 minutes. Cool for 5 minutes before serving hot, or leave to cool completely and serve cold.

✳ **TOFU CUSTARD** When mixing tofu with soya milk to make a custard-like filling such as this, I use a ratio of 3 parts milk to 5 parts tofu. I use firm tofu, if possible, and press a little water from it before I add the milk.

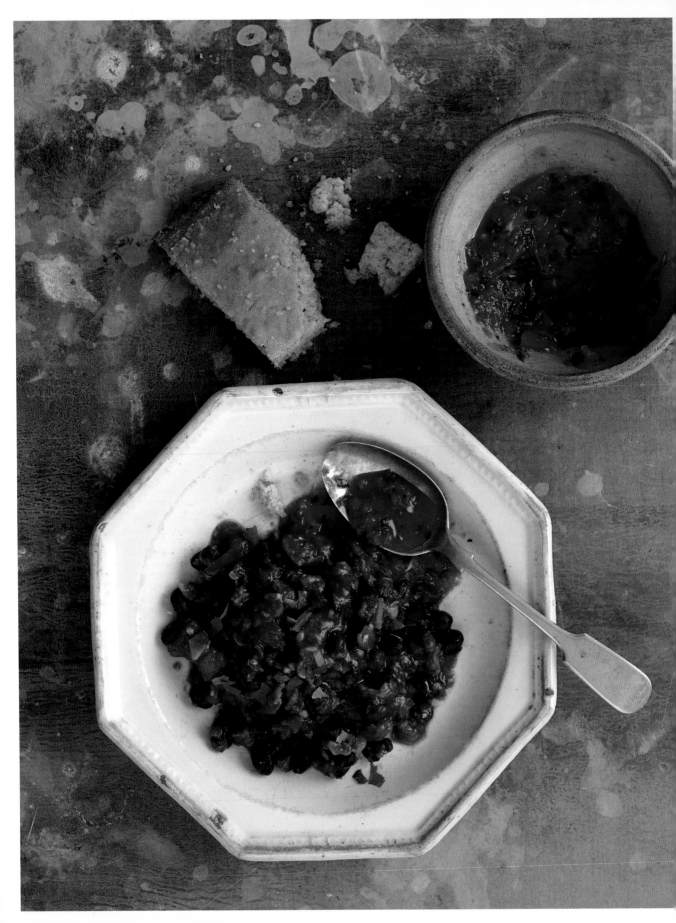

ADZUKI BEAN RAGOUT

Rich in protein and iron, these little red beans are very easy to digest. Here, they're cooked to a soft consistency with flavoursome sautéed spices. Serve the ragout on its own in bowls, or as part of a larger meal with Warm Broccoli Salad (page 151), Eat-It-Today Cornbread (page 135) and Red Pepper and Tomato Salsa (see below).

SERVES 4

PREPARATION TIME 1 HOUR +

8 HOURS SOAKING

500g (1lb 2oz) dried adzuki beans, soaked for a minimum of 8 hours (see How to Cook Beans, page 64)

10cm (4in) strip of kombu, rinsed

1 tablespoon untoasted sesame oil

1 whole garlic bulb, cloves separated and chopped

2 tablespoons grated fresh ginger

2 spring onions (scallions), finely chopped

½ –1 teaspoon dried chilli flakes, to taste

½ teaspoon ground cinnamon

½ teaspoon ground allspice

2 medium tomatoes, finely chopped

OPTIONS AND VARIATIONS

For an even richer flavour, add 1 teaspoon vegan bouillon powder while cooking the garlic, ginger and onion.

Drain and rinse the soaked beans. Put the kombu in a large saucepan and tip the drained beans on top. Add fresh water to cover the beans to a depth of about 3cm (1¼in). Cover the pan and bring to a simmer over a medium heat.

After 20 minutes, stir the beans and add more water if needed. Cover the pan and simmer the beans a further 10–15 minutes until tender.

Meanwhile, measure the sesame oil into a small pan. Over a low to medium heat, cook the garlic, ginger and spring onions for about 5 minutes, stirring once or twice. Add the spices and stir the mixture for a minute or two. Now add the chopped tomato, cover the pan and cook for 5 minutes.

When the beans are tender, drain them and return them to their pan. Tip the spiced tomato mixture into the beans and stir to combine. Keeping the pan over a low heat, add up to 100ml (3½fl oz/scant ½ cup) water, if needed, to achieve a thick ragout: a rich, spicy sauce with some whole beans and some that have lost their form.

Cover the pan and remove from the heat. Serve immediately, or leave for a couple of hours to allow the flavours to blend and mature. The ragout is good served hot or cold.

RED PEPPER AND TOMATO SALSA For a spicy accompaniment to beans or cornbread, quarter 2 red sweet peppers (capsicums) and cut away the stalk, seeds and white membranes. Grill (broil) the peppers, skin side up, until the skins begin to blister and slightly char, about 5 minutes. Cool the peppers slightly, then peel the skins away as best you can and roughly chop the flesh. Put into a blender or processor with a pinch of salt, the juice of 2 limes and 2 tablespoons extra virgin olive oil. Chop 2 fresh red chillies (deseeded if you prefer a milder salsa), 4 medium tomatoes, 6 garlic cloves, 1 small onion and 10g (¼oz/about 1 cup) coriander (cilantro) leaves, and add them to the peppers. Blend briefly to give a chunky, rough-textured salsa (don't overdo it or you'll end up with a purée). Chill the salsa for a couple of hours before serving, to allow the flavours to merge. Store in a closed container in the refrigerator for 2–3 days.

SWEETCORN AND PEPPER RELISH

This is best made from fresh sweetcorn; simply slice it from the cob after the cob has been boiled. The kernels come away in wide panels that add extra texture and appeal to this dish. A large spoonful on the side of the plate makes the perfect spicy accompaniment to a Quick Patty Cake Mix burger (page 50), Onion, Tofu and Tomato Tart (page 131) or Eat-It-Today Cornbread (page 135).

SERVES 4

PREPARATION TIME 20 MINUTES + CHILLING

2 sweetcorn cobs

2 tablespoons untoasted sesame oil

4 garlic cloves, finely chopped

1 small onion, diced

1 fresh chilli, finely chopped

1 small apple, grated

2 medium tomatoes, finely chopped

3 tablespoons finely chopped flat-leaf parsley

Pinch of ground cinnamon

Juice of 1 lime

OPTIONS AND VARIATIONS

Add fresh coriander (cilantro) instead of parsley, or use a mixture of parsley and coriander.

Preheat the oven to 200°C (400°F).

Bring a large pan of water to a rapid boil. Add the corn cobs and cook them for 8–10 minutes until tender. The colour of the kernels will change from pale yellow to golden. Lift the cobs from the water and allow to cool slightly before slicing off the corn kernels.

Put the kernels in a roasting pan with the oil, garlic and onion. Toss briefly so that everything is coated in oil, then roast in the oven for 15 minutes.

Remove from the oven and add the remaining ingredients to the roasting pan. Stir the ingredients together for about 2 minutes, then turn the relish into a serving dish.

Serve immediately or chill the relish before serving. Use within 2 days.

EAT-IT-TODAY CORNBREAD

Cornmeal tastes and behaves very differently from wheat flour. It comes in fine, medium or coarse grinds. This bread uses the fine grind, but you could use a medium grind as well. Cornbread is best eaten fresh from the oven. Try it with a spicy tomato sauce such as Red Pepper and Tomato Salsa (page 133) or with Adzuki Bean Ragout (page 133) and Precious Greens (page 193).

SERVES 4

PREPARATION TIME 40 MINUTES

100g (3½oz/⅔ cup) fine cornmeal

100g (3½oz/⅔ cup) plain (all-purpose) flour

2 teaspoon cream of tartar

1 teaspoon bicarbonate of soda (baking soda)

2 tablespoons untoasted sesame oil, plus extra for oiling the pan

200ml (7fl oz/scant 1 cup) plant milk

2 teaspoons apple cider vinegar

OPTIONS AND VARIATIONS

Add 2 tablespoons chopped fresh chives and ¼ teaspoon black pepper to the flour mixture. For a slightly crusty base to this bread, heat the oiled pan before you add the batter.

Preheat the oven to 200°C (400°F), and oil a 23 × 23cm (9 × 9in) square cake pan. Pop the pan in the oven while it is heating up (this will help the cornbread to cook quickly and evenly).

Meanwhile, mix together the cornmeal, flour, cream of tartar and bicarbonate of soda in a large bowl.

In a measuring jug (large measuring cup), stir together the oil, milk and vinegar. Working swiftly now, tip the wet mixture into the dry ingredients and stir as briefly as possible, while ensuring that everything is thoroughly and evenly mixed.

Pour the batter into the hot cake pan and bake for 15–20 minutes until the bread is golden. It will rise and its surface will crack open slightly. A skewer or the tip of a sharp knife inserted into the centre should come out clean.

Cool briefly in the pan, then cut into squares and serve warm.

POTATO AND SPINACH HOT SALAD

I have specified Pink Fir Apple potatoes because they hold their firm texture and take up other flavours without losing their slightly sweet yet earthy taste – but you can use any waxy salad potato. The spinach softens but keeps its tangy flavour. This is delicious served alongside Fresh Borlotti Bean Salad (page 104) or Tempeh Crisps in Pomegranate Glaze (page 167).

SERVES 4

PREPARATION TIME 40 MINUTES

300g (10½oz) Pink Fir Apple potatoes, cut into 1cm (½in) thick rounds

100g (3½oz/2 cups) fresh baby spinach

1 small red onion, quartered and thinly sliced

2 tablespoons untoasted sesame oil

6 garlic cloves, finely chopped

½ teaspoon caraway seeds, slightly crushed

¼ teaspoon black pepper

¼ teaspoon ground nutmeg

2 tablespoons apple cider vinegar

OPTIONS AND VARIATIONS

Use 1 tablespoon rice vinegar or lemon juice and 1 tablespoon apple cider vinegar. If you can find fresh dandelions, finely chop 20g (¾oz) dandelion leaves and cook with the garlic for 2 minutes before proceeding.

Pour water into a saucepan to a depth of 3cm (1¼in). Fit a steamer basket over the water and set the pan over a medium heat. Put the potato slices in the steamer basket and cover the pan. Steam the potatoes until tender, about 15 minutes.

Meanwhile, mix the spinach and red onion in a large serving dish and set aside.

Pour the oil into a small frying pan (skillet) set over a low heat. Add the garlic and caraway seed and cover the pan. Cook for about 5 minutes, stirring from time to time. Add the pepper and nutmeg, stir well and remove the pan from the heat.

Turn the steamed potatoes into the hot frying pan, and stir so that the potatoes absorb the flavours. Immediately tip the hot potato mixture into the serving dish and toss together with the spinach and red onion.

While the frying pan is still hot, add the vinegar and swirl it around to combine with any remaining juices. Drizzle the vinegar over the hot salad, toss again and serve.

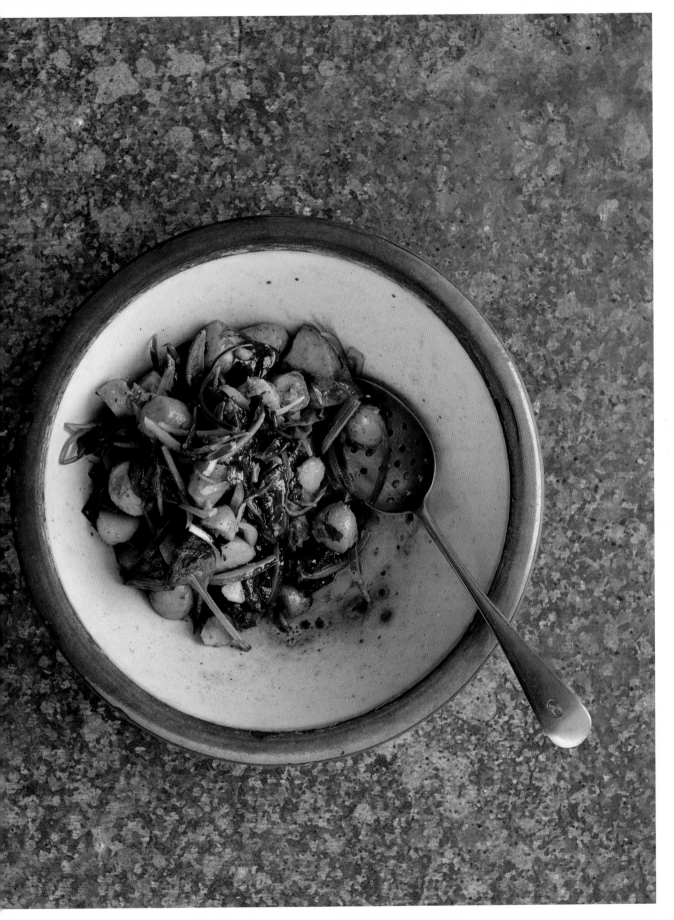

FAMILY MATTERS

EATING FOR TWO

At a time when everyone and their neighbour's uncle wants to offer advice, the most stabilizing approach is to keep it simple. By following a few basic steps, it's possible to have a healthy, happy pregnancy while on a plant-based diet. Whether you're vegan or not, the basics are really, really important during this time. Women should try to keep exercising, get 30 minutes of sunshine (or sunlight) each day, stay hydrated, rest often and eat a nutrient-rich diet.

The old adage 'eating for two' is often misinterpreted – it doesn't mean that you have to double your calorie intake or the size of food portions! It means that you need to eat responsibly to provide ample high-quality nutrients to help keep you and your baby well. The vegan diet is a natural match for this goal when you eat a variety of whole foods that are in season where you live. Eat to acquire nutrients and sufficient calories, using supplements carefully and only if necessary. Learn about four key nutrients that need your special attention – preferably before you become pregnant. They are folate, B_{12}, iron and calcium (see pages 22–25).

It is common, in the first few weeks of pregnancy, to be drawn to certain foods, such as carbohydrates or high-protein foods. These and other cravings are natural, but it is best if you meet them with a healthy food option.

* Pasta, brown rice, porridge or a plate of roasted root vegetables are all excellent sources of carbohydrates, especially appealing dressed with flaxseed or olive oil.
* Add beans or lentils, nuts or seeds, and miso, tofu or tempeh for extra protein.
* Smoothies such as Avocado Almond Shake (page 68) can provide sustaining, easy-to-digest combinations of fruit, vegetables and mineral-rich plant milks.

Queasiness or morning sickness can be soothed by:

* a plain rice cracker or oatcake
* a bowl of noodles in miso broth
* a slice of fresh ginger steeped in hot water

Snack-sized meals can be the most comfortable option in later pregnancy, when it feels like there is no room in your abdomen for a meal!

* Travel with a carton of mixed nuts and dried fruit, and a packet of crispy nori strips.
* Keep a bowl of prepared raw vegetables (crudités) in the refrigerator.
* Make nutritious dips such as Great Guacamole (page 73) or Tahini Lemon Whip (page 83).
* Have a bowl of Certainty Soup (page 155) or Dressed Greens and Beans (page 154) each day.
* Fresh fruit is nature's snack-sized meal; or try All-Seasons Fruit Salad (page 36).

Prepare for your pregnancy by upgrading your diet, now, to one that is nutrient-rich; your pregnancy and the postnatal year will be more comfortable and healthy as a result.

THE FIRST MEAL

Imagine there was one thing you could do that would begin to protect your infant from illness and allergy within hours of their birth, and then for the whole of their life. This same act would help to prevent obesity, dental cavities, viral and bacterial infections, gastric disorders and possibly type 2 diabetes. It would help your child to develop speech because of its effect on jaw, teeth and facial development, and would gift them with emotional and physical security. Imagine this act would also reduce your risks of suffering cancers of the breast, ovaries, uterus or cervix. That it helped you to lose your pregnancy weight and transformed stress to create a calm connection with your baby and a loving atmosphere in the home. Well, it's not a dream. It's called breastfeeding and it is credited with all of those benefits, and more besides.

The World Health Organization gives clear guidance, advising that: 'Infants should be breastfed exclusively during the first six months of life [and] … continuously until 2 years of age and beyond.' It also states that breastfeeding 'fosters healthy growth and improves cognitive development'. Government and health organizations from member countries echo this guidance, confirming that breast milk is sufficient and the 'ideal source of nutrition for the infant'. One study suggests that a 'scaling up of breastfeeding to a near universal level could prevent 823,000 annual deaths in children younger than 5 years and 20,000 annual deaths from breast cancer'.

From the middle term of your pregnancy and in the hours and days following birth, your body produces colostrum, a highly concentrated sort of milk that is rich in nutrients and immunity-enhancing substances. When you put your baby to the breast a short time after birth, this first meal will fill their stomach and instantly begin to protect them against germs that populate your immediate environment. The baby's suckling will signal to your body that other natural processes should begin, including the continued production of milk. Over the next few days, the colostrum is gradually replaced by a thinner milk, and as the weeks pass this milk changes slightly in composition, depending on what the baby needs. It will continue to provide all the nutrition your baby needs for the first six months of life.

In addition to its health benefits, breastfeeding is often the easiest option. Breast milk is available at the right temperature, anywhere and at any time. There is no fuss with mixing and warming formula, sterilizing bottles or packing supplies. Plus, it's free. It also helps mothers to deepen their bond and to learn to read their baby's signals and expressions months before they are able to speak.

If you decide to breastfeed, a few practical adjustments are necessary.

* You will have to be available to your infant 24/7 for the first few months.
* That doesn't mean that you can't have breaks – they will just need to be carefully arranged.
* It doesn't mean that you won't sleep, but sometimes you will fall asleep with your baby sleeping beside you.

* Think ahead and plan for regular support; it will make all the difference.
* You might want to adjust what you wear so that you can feed your baby without total exposure.
* I carried a large chiffon scarf around with me which folded into the size of a small envelope. If my baby wanted feeding, I draped the scarf over my shoulders in a way that looked fashionable but that also kept my baby-on-the-breast private. My babies could peer through the colours to see my face, and so they never tried to pull the scarf away. To this day, my children recognize the scarf when I take it out.
* You might need to maintain your resolve if friends, family or colleagues disapprove of your decision to breastfeed.
* Stay committed! You are right; they are behind the times. Humans are meant to breastfeed.
* The discouragement to breastfeed is inspired by unreasonable social and commercial pressures.
* Most medical and scientific bodies are in support of long-term breastfeeding, as already outlined, above.

I was vegan throughout my pregnancies and had very big babies. I was able to breastfeed both of them and lost all my 'pregnancy weight' after just three months' breastfeeding – I also got to eat bowls of pasta just before bed as breastfeeding uses up the calories! At six months, I found that my baby was more satisfied after I had eaten brown rice. So, for a few months, I cooked 500g (1lb 2oz/about 2½ cups) organic brown rice every morning and ate it in small meals over the course of the day. I topped it with greens, seeds or seaweed, and a tiny spoonful of miso. A dish that really made a difference to the quantity of milk I produced was Tahini Lemon Whip (page 83). I made this often, adding various ingredient options, and found it a tremendous boost to my energy levels – just what I needed to keep up with the little one! When he was about seven months, he slapped his hand into my plate, licked his palm and has loved the dish himself ever since.

DONOR MILK AND FORMULA

If, for some reason, a woman is unable to breastfeed, that is sad but also manageable. Mothers are sometimes unable to produce milk if their baby is born prematurely, but the baby can still benefit from breast milk. Pre-term or sick babies are often recipients of donor milk, which is pasteurized and the donor screened before the milk is shared. Sometimes the mother is able to hand-express a little milk each day and might, eventually, provide her own milk for the baby. Infant formula is another option for a baby whose mother is unable to nurse, for whatever reason. Formula has been available for several decades and was developed to deal with emergency situations. Controversially, its use has become commonplace in recent years. It is available in dairy- and soya-based forms.

WEANING AND TEETHING

Weaning is a gradual process that should happen alongside breastfeeding at first. It can start very casually, just dipping your finger into your own food as you eat and letting your baby taste your finger. Then, from about six months (when your baby can sit and pick up a small item of food by themselves), prop them in a high chair and offer a spoonful of mashed fruit or vegetable, or something from your own plate. You'll find your baby will want to play with it, spit it out, smear it everywhere, will want or not want it, will hold it, throw it, drop it and sometimes hide it in their clothing. Take your time and enjoy this phase. Babies need time to learn how to eat solid foods! Keep your camera ready because this is a time of great photo opportunities – a joyous but extremely messy phase.

Plant-based food is ideal for weaning: it is natural, full of nutrients and easy to digest. Here are some tips on how to start:

* Start with mashed foods such as avocado, banana or cooked carrot; or soft foods such as apple purée (without the peel) or well-cooked red lentils. Rice flakes cooked in rice or almond milk make an excellent first porridge. A little Plum Butter (page 45) can be stirred in or served on its own. Feed with a spoon or offer this food in an open cup or bowl, and let your baby use their fingers to feed themselves. You can give them a baby spoon, but it might not be used for its intended purpose.
* Next, offer large chunks of cooked food that they can easily hold, such as a stalk of steamed broccoli or a wedge of steamed, peeled sweet potato. Make sure cooked foods are cooled first and are tender enough to easily fall apart in the baby's mouth.
* Later, offer foods that need chewing. This is partly to let them explore the texture in their mouth and also to help them to learn the chewing technique. Try a few strands of cooled spaghetti, a chunk of peeled banana or a small bowl of peeled and grated apple. Flaked rice or oat flakes (rolled oats) cooked into a thin porridge are also foods they can feed to themselves.

There are a few key things to keep in mind as you introduce solid foods to your baby:

* Stay close and pay attention to avoid a risk of your baby choking.
* Avoid foods that are high in salt or sugar, and don't add sweeteners or salt to the foods you prepare for them.
* Avoid foods with a risk of allergy for your baby's first year of life. The foods that most commonly cause allergies in children are eggs, milk (all types, including formula), soya, wheat (gluten) and peanuts.
* Soya is a high-protein food that your infant might not be ready to digest for a year or two. Oat or rice milk is a good alternative liquid to mix with their porridge, for instance. Otherwise, water remains the best drink, as well as breast milk.
* A little wheat, such as the end of a baguette, is okay to gnaw when they start teething. However, greatly limit the amount you offer for at least the first year.

* Peanuts and peanut butter are best introduced slowly after the fourth year.

Breastfeeding will reduce as baby grows and derives more of their nourishment from the foods you offer, but not at first and not all at once.

TEETHING

This is the definition of misery! Imagine, your skull starts to re-form, forcing bony spikes through the skin inside your mouth. You are aching, feverish, sick to your stomach from the pain, can't sleep properly, and there's a strange itchiness that makes you just want to … bite!

Teething happens over and over again until early adulthood. The depth of misery depends on the age and disposition of the young person, but it's not nice. These simple ideas can help:

* Gnawing foods help, but which you choose will depend on the age of your young person.

* The rounded end of a baguette is hard enough to take the drool and gnawing of an infant for quite some time. Messy though it may be, it will soothe.

* Toast thick slices of Splendid Wholesome Loaf (page 120) in a low-heat oven. Remove the soft middle part and let your infant gnaw on the dry crusts.

* Raw carrot is excellent for older children, who will not choke on the small pieces of carrot they gnaw away.

* Make a double-strength cup of chamomile tea (two teabags per cup) and let it cool. Serve this to infants in spoonfuls or in their little mugs. Older children can enjoy 2–3 cups per day.

* For older children, make their favourite ice lollies (popsicles) and let them have any number of them. The cold can help to soothe their discomfort. See Epic Ice Lollies (page 81).

GROWING PAINS

Here are some of the hurdles every parent will have to encounter at some point in their child's development.

GROWTH SPURTS

Developmental growth can coincide with a physical growth spurt, and it makes sense to link them. During these periods, your child might get grumpy, clumsy and unfocused, and lose interest in their usual favourite foods. They might prefer a high-calorie mono-diet or protein-rich foods and lots of them. Take the hint and provide what they need, but aim for variation and nutrition, not just empty calories.

* Mineral-rich foods are essential, especially considering that new bone is being built.
* Good sources are crispy seaweed, hummus, bean butters, whole grains and greens.
* For leg pains: make Miso and Tahini Protein-Booster Sandwich (page 123). Squeeze lemon juice into water to drink this after eating the sandwich.
* High-calorie food is best from complex carbohydrates rather than simple sugars.
* A falafel wrap, a plate of rice and beans, or a bowl of Barley and Oat Groat Porridge (page 56) will give slow-release support, in preference to desserts, pastries and biscuits (cookies).
* For an instant-sugar requirement, fresh or dried fruit is always best.
* Protein is abundant in a varied vegan diet. A daily serving of beans or lentils, tofu or tempeh, and nuts or seeds will provide significant amounts.
* For a protein boost, stir 1 teaspoon spirulina or chlorella into a large glass of plant milk (try almond or oat milk), and whisk together. These milks are mineral-rich and the powders are protein-rich, making this a highly nutritious snack.
* Mushrooms are rich in vitamin D, which supports the immune system and helps to build bone. Basic requirements for vitamin D can be met by getting regular exercise outdoors, in the daylight. Vitamin D and exercise are a good combination for enhancing mood as well.

ILLNESS

I can think of two good things about being ill: realizing someone cares and, later, the amazing zest for life that surges through you when you start to feel better. If you are caring for a sick child, here are a few things you can feed them that will aid recovery:

* The BRAT diet is famous the world over – at least, it is once you've heard about it. It stands for Banana, Rice, Apple juice and dry Toast. These are simple foods that provide a range of useful nutrients, usually without causing additional upset.
* Herbal teas can help to soothe and hydrate. Put 1–2 teaspoons of herb into a cup or small teapot, and add boiling water:

- Yarrow to help break a fever (add a little barley malt syrup if this is too bitter)
- Thin slices (4-6) of fresh ginger to ease a cough or sore throat
- Lime blossom or chamomile to help get off to sleep

✳ A simple broth in a cup will help to raise energy levels and fight infection:
  - Pour not-quite-boiling water over 2 garlic cloves, a pinch of cayenne pepper and ¼ teaspoon miso. Stir well and leave to steep for 10 minutes. Sip from cup or spoon.
  - See also All-Nations Onion Soup (page 152) and Lettuce and Ginger Broth (page 89).

After they have 'turned the corner' and are starting to feel better, offer these:

✳ Divine Popcorn (page 67) is life-affirming and helps to bind in the case of diarrhoea.

✳ Pasta drizzled with olive oil and 2 tablespoons almond milk is a simple, warming meal that feeds recovery and stimulates the appetite without upsetting the digestion.

✳ Rehydration is crucial. Stir 1 teaspoon barley malt syrup, a pinch of sea salt and the juice of ½ lemon into a tall glass of water. Offer this again in an hour.

✳ Mineral-rich blackstrap molasses gives a dose of lost nutrients. Stir 1 teaspoon molasses into a half-cup of boiled water. Leave to cool until just warm, then sip.

BIG SULKS

These can happen at any age. You don't need to know the reason – in fact, sometimes they don't know the reason. Sulks can be useful provided they don't go on for too long. They allow the sulker to experience life 'from the outside' because, being sulky, they don't want to join in and other people don't necessarily want them to, either!

If a bit of time and space don't seem to be working, try some of these:

✳ For very young people, a sulk may be transformed quite effectively by giving them a sink full of water to play with. Alternatively, put them in water, such as a bath or paddling pool. Stay close, but let them splash it out.

✳ Slightly older young people often emerge from their gloom when they are given a big challenge, a new responsibility or … a cookery project.

✳ A sulk in any age group will be eased by making a 'vineberry' drink. This is 2 teaspoons each of apple cider vinegar and berry juice (any berry) stirred into an 240ml (8fl oz) glass of water. Some people even ask for more vinegar!

✳ Include Barley and Oat Groat Porridge (page 56) in their diet for a few days. Barley and oats are nutrient-dense complex carbohydrates that will provide a slow-release supply of energy. These grains also can create a calm steadiness that helps the sulker to move into a better frame of mind.

✳ Make sure that they are getting enough of the B group of vitamins by offering whole grains, beans and lentils, nuts, seeds and yeast products.

THE TWO-MEAL FAMILY

So your daughter has just announced that she has 'gone vegan'. Or your son's partner is pregnant and they plan to raise the child on a vegan diet. Or, perhaps you have decided to eat a vegan diet, but your partner is not so keen. How can it possibly work?

Stay calm: these situations are increasingly common and needn't be a problem. It's okay to be part of a two-meal family! Good communication and a few practical changes will help you to integrate everyone's dietary needs into your family meals.

ROUND TABLE

It is easy for individuals to assume that because they have found a way of living that suits them, they are right and the other is wrong. That they are better than the other, or more intelligent, more sensitive, more relevant … These assumptions really do not help! Pressure, disapproval and self-righteousness can become toxic.

If you are the omnivore, remember that everyone has their own point of view. If a person does not act – or is prevented from acting – in support of their individuality, the real problems start to mount up. Be brave and open up a dialogue:

* Let them explain how they came to their decision and really listen. You have a choice: be adversarial and judgmental, or be open to all that is potentially positive about their choice and decide to make it work between you.
* Discover what you can learn *from* them: for example, some delicious new recipes.
* Learn about some aspect of the diet *with* them: for example, nutrition, cooking techniques, new ingredients.
* Take the initiative: find a vegan cooking class or café you can attend together.
* Consider the possibility they are doing the right thing and try it with them!

If you are the vegan in the situation, pull back and do some clear thinking:

* You might want them to adopt a plant-based diet with you, but if it was the other way around you wouldn't appreciate pressure or disapproval from them.
* Be patient. They might wish to make the switch at some point in the future.
* Everyone has their own inner 'timer'. Just because you are eager to make this change now, doesn't mean they have to be.
* Your loved one is more likely to join you in your new way of eating if you create an atmosphere of respectful acceptance, rather than intolerance – but you can try to lure them with delicious vegan dinners!

Stay committed to your loved one, nurture harmony and respect, keep talking, keep hugging and negotiate changes together. Aim for 'small' solutions and allow plenty of time for each change to settle in. This takes the pressure off everyone. In the early days, most changes and negotiations involve practicalities to do with shopping for food, eating out, storage of food and who does the cooking.

WHO COOKS?

You might assume that the cook gets to make all the decisions. That can work, but it is a tad controlling and, in this situation, could cause trouble. If you are the cook:

* Agree to reduce the number of times per week that meat is cooked
* Agree to make your partner's usual favourites but using vegan ingredients

If you and your partner both cook, but one of you doesn't want to cook meat:

* Agree that meat items are cooked by the person who eats them
* Agree that your omnivore eats meat when out for a meal but not at home
* Agree that both of you will sample look-alike foods until you each find favourites

If you are cooking for a newly vegan member of your family:

* Agree you will take turns making the family meals
* Agree to share new skills, new recipes, new ingredients
* Agree to go shopping for food together

SWAP SHOPPING

Like it or not, most people have grown up on a meat and two veg diet, which creates an expectation as to what a meal looks like. Corporate food producers are responding to the increasing consumer demand for plant-based foods and now provide many plant-based 'meat replacements'. This is a useful product group.

Not everyone feels the need for these products, but there are good reasons to see what is available. Substitutes can sometimes take the pressure off a family member who has not yet chosen to eat a vegan diet. If the look-alike is tasty and holds the expected position on the plate, they might decide animal-derived foods are not necessary after all.

The occasional purchase of such food items sends the right message to the producers: that there is a steady and growing demand for plant-based food products. For vegans, it can feel like a treat to 'test drive' a new plant milk, non-dairy ice cream or vegan cheese. You can try using plant-based cutlets, bean burgers and various styles of sausages as substitutes in your family's favourite meals.

KITCHEN ETIQUETTE

Excuse the pun, but kitchen etiquette can really stir things up! Keep it simple: if you don't want animal-derived foods to be cooked in the pans you use for vegan meals, buy another set of pans and designate which is which.

If you don't want animal-derived foods to be stored in the refrigerator or freezer, you need to agree boundaries. For example, you may be comfortable with one carton of dairy milk being stored for your partner's tea, and agreeing that meat products are used on the day of purchase. Alternatively, you could request that no animal-derived food is to be brought into the home. These issues can be solved if you talk about them openly.

WHAT TO SERVE WHEN THEY BRING THEIR FRIENDS HOME

When your children bring friends over, the first rule is that whatever you serve must look 'normal'. It helps if it also looks like a treat and (here is the second rule) there must be lots of it. You will be lucky if you learn ahead of time that there will be visitors, for that would allow you time to prepare! More likely, you will be descended upon and (the third rule) you will be lovingly expected to provide a table full of provisions quickly and then disappear.

   All of this requires some kitchen management, a lot of patience and more than a little thinking ahead. Here are some ideas that might help:

* Open a packet of store-bought wraps and put out bowls of ingredients for them to choose from: sliced cucumber, grated carrot, hummus, mustard and ketchup, olives, chopped lettuce and tomatoes, sliced pickles and some freshly warmed falafel. Then leave them to it unless they specifically ask how to fold or roll the wrap. (They won't.)
* Fill a number of small bowls with salsa, hummus, guacamole and relish. Serve a plate laden with fruit and vegetable crudités. Don't stand there and watch, and absolutely do not encourage them to try the fresh food. (They will.)
* Open your cupboard and pull out everything that could possibly be seen as a spread: peanut butter, yeast extract, jams, miso, brown sauce, pesto, bean butter, tahini and sriracha sauce. Put everything on the table. Hand around plates and table knives, point to the loaf of bread and put your own child in charge of the toaster.
* If you know they are coming, you can make pie. Sweet or savoury, flans or pasties, all pie forms are life-enhancing to young people. You are allowed to slice and lift the first piece, after which you must hand the spatula to one of them. It's okay to point out the location of the dustpan and brush as you depart for another room. It's not okay to say, 'Do it properly.'
* You might occasionally go the route of providing cookies, cakes or bars. If they let you in the kitchen, you can cook them there and then for that freshly baked experience. However, you must pretend you're not listening to their conversation.
* Remember that carob looks and tastes like chocolate. Use the syrup to make 'chocolate' milkshakes, the powder to make 'chocolate' cakes and cookies, the spread to make 'chocolate' wraps and pizzas. Carob is naturally sweet, caffeine-free and calcium-rich.
* Add the juice of a freshly squeezed lemon and orange to a jug (pitcher) of sparkling water for a natural fizzy drink.
* Finally, popcorn is a whole grain so it's almost a health food! But don't tell anyone.

This phase of life goes on for some time, so you might as well get sorted. If you have a freezer, devote a section of it to food that will light up these social occasions and free you from a feeling of panic at being caught unprepared.

BEFORE THEY LEAVE HOME

It is a wise young person who learns to cook before they leave home. Here are twelve types of dish that will set them up for good. With a repertoire such as this, who could ever go hungry, become bored or be found inhospitable?

SOUP The rule for making a great soup is you should not be able to taste the water. Add twice the number of onions you think are necessary; they will produce a deep background flavour. Simple soups to begin with are White Bean Soup (page 205) and Sorrel Soup (page 170).

SALAD DRESSING A good dressing can unify the various flavours in a salad to change it from good to exquisite. Make an emulsion by shaking or stirring together 1 part vinegar, some chopped herbs, salt, mustard or spices, and 3 parts oil.

GRAIN When you know How to Cook Whole Grains (see page 60), you can create a whole meal – just by adding herbs and spices, vegetables and beans.

STEW A one-pot meal that takes all the vegetables you can give to it! Call it a curry or casserole, it can feed any number of flatmates and is great for breakfast, too. Great ones to know are Homecoming Stew (page 204) and Chickpea and Ruby Chard Hubbub (page 198).

STIR-FRY Quick and dramatic; prepare the vegetables in advance so that, when the cooking starts, they can be added in rapid sequence. Heat the pan, then add cold oil, then vegetables. Try Stir-Fried Vegetables over Spiced Noodles (page 114).

ROAST DINNER Impressive, welcoming and easy to make. The biggest hurdle is getting everything to be ready at the same time. Don't forget the gravy. Try Roast Dinner Medley (page 175) and Gravy of the Gods (page 208).

LEFTOVERS An art form! Jazz up with fresh ingredients to make Bubble 'n' Squeak (page 53) or re-purpose with a sauce or side dish.

PIE A tart, a pasty or a full double-crust mountain of pie can make the world right again. Aim to know one fruit and one savoury version. I'd recommend Blueberry Apple Pie (page 216) and Onion, Tofu and Tomato Tart (page 131).

CAKE It's always a celebration; it doesn't always need icing! My fail-safe starter recipe is Old-Fashioned Seed Cake (page 84).

COOKIES Quick to make with basic ingredients – great to share at work or uni (college). The Chocolate Chip Cookies (page 96) always go down well.

BREAD An ancient craft, totally hands-on with exquisite aromas and infinite versions possible. Learn the basics first (try Splendid Wholesome Loaf on page 120), then start adding herbs, spices, fruits and seeds.

DRINKS Aim for a tisane, a plant-milky hot drink, a smoothie. These would be my top choices – Iced Midsummer Tisane (page 82), Choc Hotlate (page 171) and Avocado Almond Shake (page 68).

SIMPLE SUPPERS

WARM BROCCOLI SALAD

This dish is quick and sustaining, colourful and tasty – perfect for when you want all the goodness of a salad but need a little warmth, too. Serving this warm really brings out the flavours of the raw ingredients. Use this as a filling for a baked potato, or to accompany Seaweed and Potato Cutlets (page 206) or Scalloped Potato Bake (page 189). If you don't finish it straight away, it is delicious cold, too, especially next to Yellow Rice Zinger (page 129).

SERVES 4

PREPARATION TIME 20 MINUTES

1 head of broccoli (600g/1lb 5oz), florets quartered

1 small carrot, grated

1 small courgette (zucchini), cut into matchsticks

1 small red onion, quartered and thinly sliced

1 apple, finely chopped

2 tablespoons chopped fresh basil

50g (1¾oz/about ½ cup) crushed walnuts

Velvet Vinaigrette (page 246)

OPTIONS AND VARIATIONS

Use 50g (1¾oz/about ½ cup) crushed hazelnuts instead of the walnuts, and add ¼ teaspoon ground cinnamon.

Arrange the broccoli florets in a basket steamer. Pour water to a depth of about 3cm (1¼in) into a saucepan, fit the steamer basket into the pan, cover and cook over a medium heat for 10–12 minutes.

Meanwhile, mix together the remaining ingredients in a serving bowl.

When the broccoli is tender but still bright green, lift out the basket and tip the broccoli in with the other ingredients.

Gently stir the salad so that all the components are evenly distributed and dressed in the vinaigrette. Serve warm.

ALL-NATIONS ONION SOUP

I really do think that food is a delicious medicine. The whole of the onion family of plants is good for the lungs and for fighting off infections. At the first hint that any one of my family has a cold, or if they're simply tired and rather lacklustre, I prepare a large pot of this soup. It has a slight sweetness, enhanced by the parsnip and the spices. Any and all members of the onion family can be added. Serve with toast, made from Splendid Wholesome Loaf (page 120) or Seeded Spelt Bread (page 87).

SERVES 4

PREPARATION TIME 40 MINUTES

1 tablespoon untoasted sesame oil

1 medium parsnip, diced

4 large onions, chopped

1 large leek, chopped

6 garlic cloves, chopped

1 teaspoon vegan bouillon powder

½ teaspoon black pepper

¼ teaspoon ground nutmeg

1.25 litres (44fl oz/5 cups) vegetable stock or water

3 tablespoons chopped fresh basil or coriander (cilantro)

4 spring onions (scallions), finely chopped

OPTIONS AND VARIATIONS

A carrot instead of the parsnip will also add sweetness, although the soup will be a different colour. Try garnishing each serving with a pinch of cayenne pepper.

Measure the sesame oil into a large stockpot or saucepan. Put the parsnip in the bottom of the pan, followed by layers of the onions, leek and garlic, in that order. Set the pan over a medium-high heat and cook for 5 minutes. Add the bouillon powder, black pepper and nutmeg. Stir well and reduce the heat to low.

Cover the pan and let the onion mixture cook for about 20 minutes until the onions are very tender and starting to caramelize. Don't cook the onions over too high a heat, or they will brown and become crisp (which is not desirable here).

Add the stock, and purée the soup using a hand-held blender. Stir in the fresh herbs and bring the soup to a gentle simmer.

Stir in the spring onions, then remove the soup from the heat and allow to cool slightly before serving.

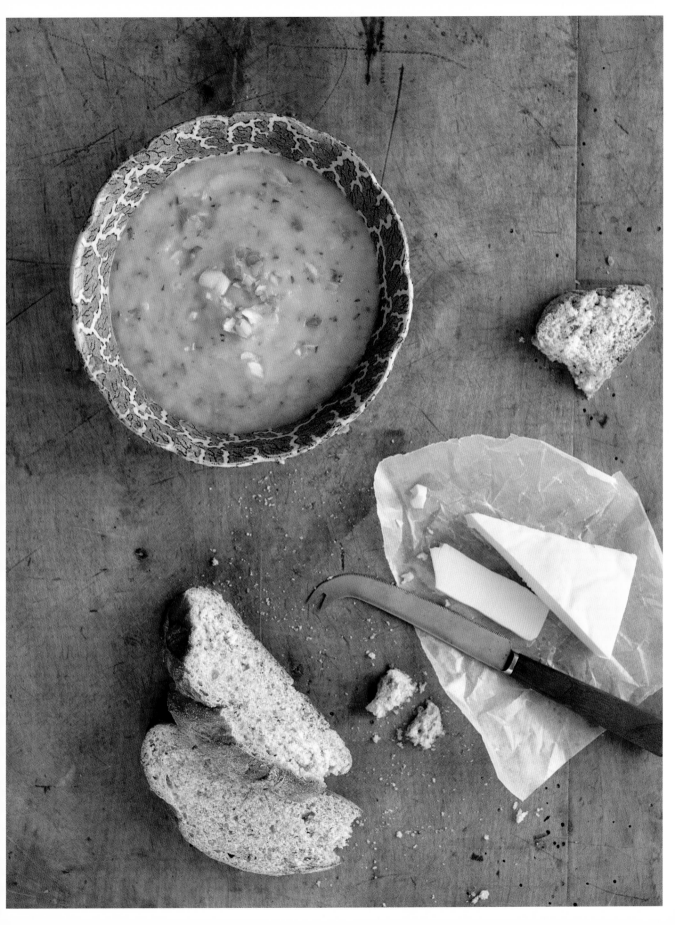

DRESSED GREENS AND BEANS

Here is possibly the simplest way of preparing and serving a generous platter of greens. Steam them for as short a time as possible, so that they retain their colour and slightly firm texture. Then don't hold back: they are full of the vitamins and minerals we all need every day. Delicious with Tempeh Crisps in Pomegranate Glaze (page 167) or Nettle and Chive Omelette (page 161).

SERVES 4

PREPARATION TIME 20 MINUTES

1 head of broccoli (about 500g/1lb), cut into florets

400g (14oz) Brussels sprouts, trimmed

400g (14oz) French (string) beans, trimmed and halved

Velvet Vinaigrette (page 244)

OPTIONS AND VARIATIONS

Use cauliflower or any type or mixture of broccoli.

Pour water into a large saucepan to a depth of 4cm (1½in). Fit a steaming basket over the water and set the pan over a medium heat. Put the broccoli, Brussels sprouts and beans into the steaming basket, and cover the pan. Steam for 10 minutes until the greens are just tender.

Transfer the vegetables to a serving dish or platter, and dress with the vinaigrette. Serve immediately – although this is also delicious cold.

CERTAINTY SOUP

I always feel that the nutritional value in this soup is certain to benefit anyone who eats it. The broth keeps all the ingredients in full view. It's easy to digest, rather more-ish and a perfect lunch or supper for an elderly person … and their grandchildren. Excellent with a thick slice of Seeded Spelt Bread (page 87).

Pour the oil into a large stockpot or saucepan set over a medium heat. Add the vegetables, nori and black pepper, and cover the pan. Leave to cook for 15 minutes, stirring once or twice in that time

Add the stock, stir and bring to a simmer. Add the tofu, and stir well. Return the soup to a simmer, then remove from the heat.

Stir in the miso paste just before serving.

SERVES 4

PREPARATION TIME 40 MINUTES

1 tablespoon untoasted sesame oil

2 celery stalks, finely chopped

1 leek, quartered along its length and finely chopped

2 tablespoons grated fresh ginger

1 whole garlic bulb, cloves separated and sliced or finely chopped

1 large carrot, grated

55g (2oz/1¾ cups) finely chopped fresh flat-leaf parsley

1 sheet of nori (such as used to wrap sushi), cut into small strips

½ teaspoon black pepper

1.5 litres (53fl oz/6 cups) vegetable stock or water

200g (7oz) firm tofu, cut into small cubes (about 1 cup prepared)

1 tablespoon miso paste

OPTIONS AND VARIATIONS

The parsley can be replaced by the same volume of thinly sliced cabbage. The miso can be replaced by a vegetable concentrate paste.

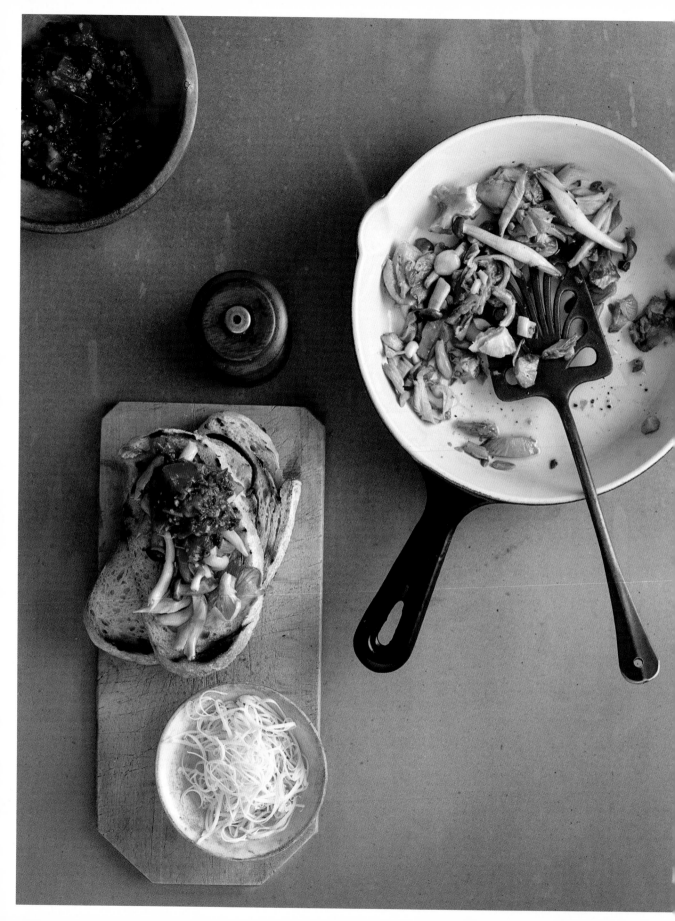

HOT MUSHROOM OPEN SANDWICH

Use your favourite mushrooms for this sandwich: I generally make this with oyster mushrooms, but I have made it with ceps (porcini), and once with a mixture that included morels. Though I call it a sandwich, it's left open and you might want to use a knife and fork to eat it. To prepare it, you'll need two pans and some very fresh bread, such as focaccia. Or try it with opened-out slices of Eat-It-Today Cornbread (page 135).

SERVES 2

PREPARATION TIME 30 MINUTES

2 tablespoons untoasted sesame oil

400g (14oz) fresh mushrooms, sliced

8 garlic cloves, chopped

55g (2oz/1¾ cups) chopped fresh flat-leaf parsley

1 medium tomato, chopped

½ teaspoon dried basil

¼ teaspoon chilli flakes

2 roughly 10cm (4in) squares of focaccia, sliced open

2 tablespoons chopped fresh basil

100g (3½oz/about 1 cup) grated vegan Cheddar-type cheese

1 tablespoon tamari

OPTIONS AND VARIATIONS

Sprinkle a pinch of ground cinnamon over the mushrooms about 5 minutes before they finish cooking.

Measure 1 tablespoon of the oil into a large frying pan (skillet) set over a medium heat. Add the mushrooms and cover the pan. Leave to cook for 10 minutes.

Pour the remaining oil into a smaller frying pan and add the garlic, parsley, tomato, basil and chilli. Cover the pan and set over a low heat.

Stir and turn the mushrooms from time to time. Your aim is to ensure that they cook evenly. Cover the pan and leave to cook for a further 10 minutes.

Stir the garlic mixture, cover the pan and leave over a very low heat until ready to serve.

Lay the bread of your choice open on the serving plates. Spoon the cooked mushrooms evenly across the open bread, then spoon the garlic mixture over the mushrooms. Sprinkle the fresh basil over the garlic mixture and grated cheese over the basil.

Add half the tamari to each pan while the frying pans are still hot. Swirl it round to collect any residual juices and pour the liquid together into one pan. Spoon this sauce over the sandwiches and serve.

✳ **MUSHROOMS** are the fruiting body of mycelium, the threadlike network of cells that live in the soil and perform the work of recycling. Mushrooms are highly nutritious and flavoursome. They store well when dried and remain a versatile addition to your meals.

OLIVE, RADICCHIO AND PASTA SALAD

I like to use bizarre or oversized pasta shapes for this salad, which is otherwise very simple. It's a perfect meal when it's late and you are weary, or when it's hot and you need something that's light but sustaining. The date molasses is a fantastic flavour companion to the bitterness of radicchio. When taking servings from the bowl, aim to take a portion from the top of the salad all the way through to the bottom of the dish where there will be a little more of the cooking juices (Is there such a thing as a vertical serving?). If you'd like extra dressing, serve with a little Herb and Garlic Drizzle (page 209).

SERVES 4

PREPARATION TIME 30 MINUTES

250g (9oz) dried pasta

2 tablespoons extra virgin olive oil, plus extra for drizzling

4 garlic cloves, finely chopped

2 spring onions (scallions), finely chopped

80g (2¾oz/about ⅔ cup) pitted olives, sliced

40g (1½oz) radicchio, sliced

3 tablespoons chopped fresh basil leaves

Juice of ½ lemon

Date molasses for drizzling

Salt and pepper, to taste

OPTIONS AND VARIATIONS

Use any type of olives you like: green or black, stuffed or not. If they come in oil, you can add the oil to the salad, too. But olive pits are a bad idea: please double-check that not a one is included. I once made this salad without basil because I didn't check first to make sure that I had it (tsk!) – chopped fresh rocket (arugula) worked very well in its place.

Set a large saucepan of water over a high heat and bring to the boil. Add the pasta and cook according to the packet instructions, until just tender.

Meanwhile, put the oil in a frying pan (skillet) set over a medium heat and add the garlic and spring onions. Stir, then cover the pan and reduce the heat to low. Cook for about 5 minutes until the onions and garlic are softened. Remove from the heat.

Drain the cooked pasta and tip into a serving dish.

Add the olives and radicchio to the garlic mixture in the pan, and stir well. Now add the basil, season with salt and pepper, and stir again.

Tip the contents of the frying pan over the cooked pasta. Pour the lemon juice into the frying pan, swirl it around to gather any residual oils and flavours, then pour this over the pasta.

Gently toss to distribute the ingredients. Leave the salad to cool or serve warm, drizzling each portion with a little olive oil and a few drops of date molasses.

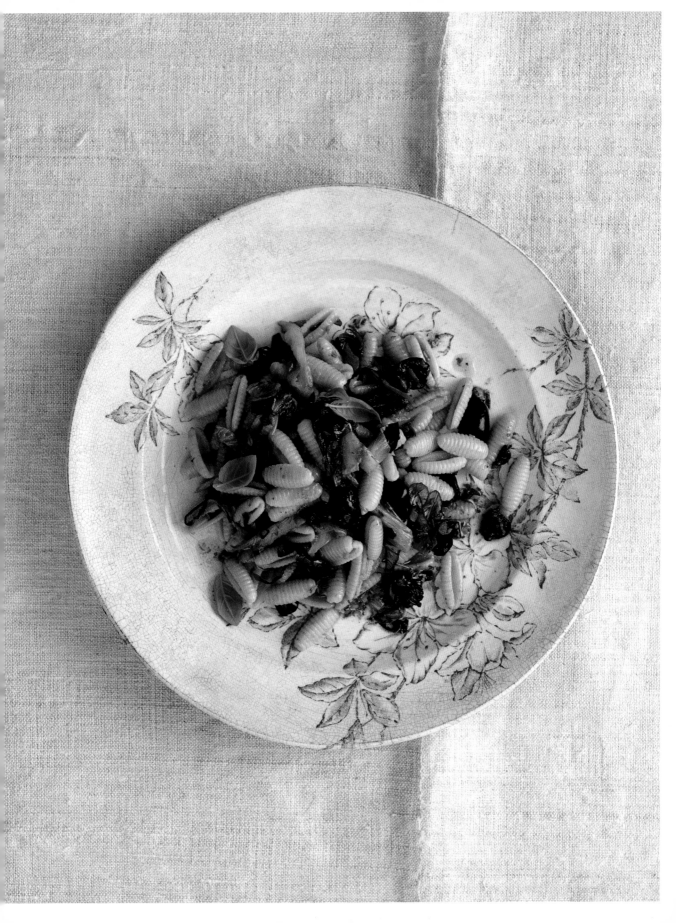

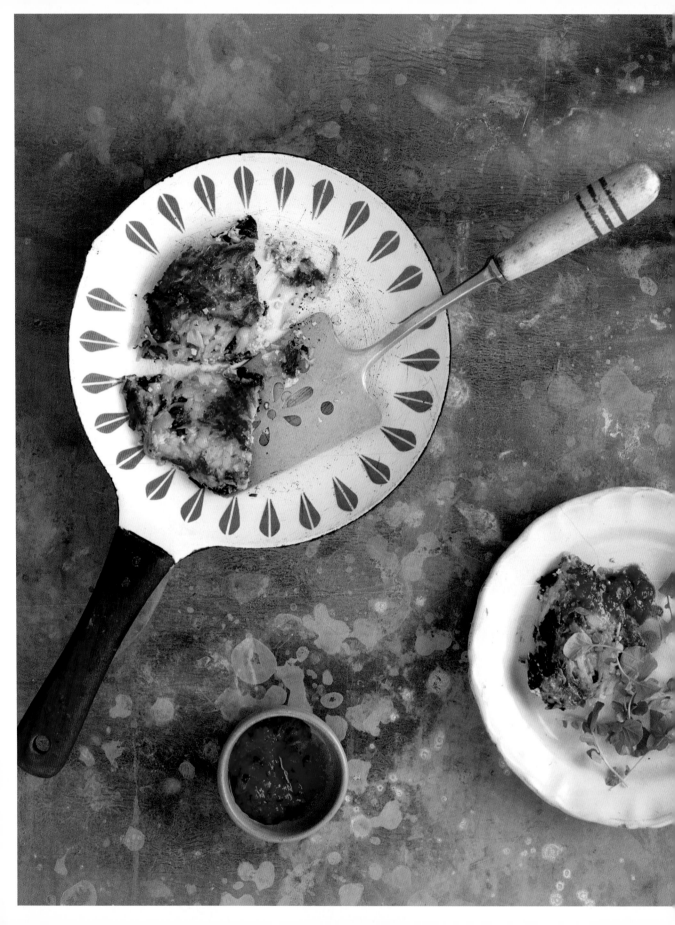

NETTLE AND CHIVE OMELETTE

I find the flavours and textures of this egg-free omelette very pleasing. I've never been very accomplished at folding and flipping hot things in a small pan, but I enjoy practising. Depending on the appetites of those at the table, sometimes an omelette of this size serves four, sometimes only two. Once, I saw one very hungry person finish the whole thing! Excellent with a little Red Pepper and Tomato Salsa (page 133).

MAKES 1 LARGE OMELETTE

PREPARATION TIME 35 MINUTES

1 tablespoons untoasted sesame oil

1 small potato, grated

2 garlic cloves, finely chopped

240g (8½oz) silken tofu, drained

3 tablespoons nutritional yeast flakes

¼ teaspoon ground turmeric

20g (¾oz) picked nettle leaves, chopped

2 tablespoons finely chopped fresh chives

Pinch of dried oregano

Salt and pepper, to taste

OPTIONS AND VARIATIONS

Use chopped sorrel or celery leaves instead of the nettles.

Put the oil into a large frying pan (skillet) set over a medium heat.

Mix the grated potato in a bowl with the garlic. Spread this mixture evenly into the frying pan and cook for 5 minutes.

Meanwhile, in a bowl, mash together the tofu, nutritional yeast flakes and turmeric. Blend the mixture together as best you can.

Sprinkle the chopped nettles and chives over the potato in the frying pan. Cover the pan and cook for 2 minutes.

Sprinkle the oregano over the greens in the pan, and season with salt and pepper. Pour over the tofu mixture, spreading it evenly. Leave to cook, uncovered, for 10 minutes. Fold the omelette in half or slice into quarters and turn each portion. Cook, uncovered, for 7–10 minutes. Serve hot.

✳ **TOFU TYPES** All tofu is not equal! Some almost pour out of their packaging, while others sit in a quivering block slowly draining water. The amount of water in your tofu can make or break a recipe, but to some extent you can work with whatever you find. Here's how. If the tofu is firm enough for you to pick up the block, hold it between your hands and gently squeeze to expel excess water (it helps if you imagine the tofu is a book that you are pressing between your palms). I've managed to squeeze up to 140ml (4½fl oz) water out of a block of tofu in this way! If the tofu is too soft to pick up, tip it into a piece of muslin (cheesecloth), tie the corners together and hang it over a bowl to let some excess water drip out. Sometimes a firm tofu is perfect but, if it is too firm, simply mash it up with a tablespoon or two of soya milk.

PIZZICATO PIZZA

Make these for a light meal or when your children unexpectedly bring friends home; or you could let them make the pizzas (while you serve as oven attendant). Messy ... but fun! The bread you select must be crusty enough to hold its shape during cooking and eating.

SERVES 4

PREPARATION TIME 30 MINUTES

8 small slices of crusty bread

160g (5¾oz) olive tapenade

1 medium courgette (zucchini), grated

200g (7oz/1⅔ cups) pitted olives, sliced

30g (1oz/½ cup) finely chopped fresh basil

2 medium tomatoes, thinly sliced

100g (3½oz/1 cup) grated vegan Mozzarella-type cheese

Salt and pepper, to taste

OPTIONS AND VARIATIONS

A pinch of dried basil sprinkled over each slice can replace the fresh basil.

Preheat the grill (broiler) until hot and lightly toast the slices of bread.

Spread a little tapenade on each piece of toast. Sprinkle grated courgette evenly over the tapenade, then arrange the sliced olives over the courgette. Next, sprinkle the chopped basil evenly over the olives, and arrange the tomato over the basil. Season with salt and pepper.

Grill (broil) for 10 minutes until the tomato is sizzling a little. Sprinkle grated cheese over each 'pizza' and grill for another 2–3 minutes.

Serve hot, but not too hot – it's best to let these stand for a minute or two, as both courgette and tomato hold their heat.

POMEGRANATE AND LEMON MARINADE

You can marinate all kinds of foods in this delicious, fruity combination. Fried tempeh and tofu are favourites; mushrooms also are a possibility, as are raw turnips and some fruits. Lift the marinated food out of the liquid to serve, but pour the marinade into a jug (pitcher) and put it on the table so you can add it as a dressing to other dishes in the meal. A little of this is nice over Dressed Greens and Beans (page 154), especially when that dish is served cold. Mop up any left on your plate with a slice of Four-day Sourdough Bread (page 118).

MAKES ABOUT 250ml (1 CUP)

PREPARATION TIME 10 MINUTES

Juice of 2 lemons

4 tablespoons pomegranate molasses

2 tablespoons tamari

2 garlic cloves, finely chopped

Pinch of cayenne pepper

OPTIONS AND VARIATIONS

Use the juice of 1 lemon mixed with 2 tablespoons apple cider vinegar. Add 4 whole cloves to the marinade.

Mix together all the ingredients in a nonreactive bowl or measuring jug (large measuring cup). Pour the mixture over cooked tempeh or tofu, or sliced raw turnips, and leave to marinate for at least 1 hour.

Refrigerate the dish if you plan to marinate it for a longer period.

✳ **HOW TO USE MARINADES** They don't always look special, but the flavours a marinade brings can make simple food very special. A marinade acts to help preserve a food as well as to add flavour to it. The preservation is made possible by the acidic ingredients, such as vinegar or lemon juice, as well as the salt which, in this recipe, is provided by the tamari. You could say that a brine, such as you find in pickles or sauerkraut, is a marinade. Spices such as chillies can also influence preservation. For vegan dishes, marinades are generally used for what they can add in terms of flavour. They are especially important when it comes to tempeh and tofu, which can otherwise seem bland. I always lightly fry these first, then slip them into a marinade, sometimes just for an hour but more often for anywhere up to 12 hours. If it's for that long, I cover them and put the dish in the refrigerator.

ROSEMARY TWIST

I love the flavour and goodness of wholemeal flours, but I'm fascinated by lighter refined flours, too. I tend to use wholemeal most of the time and enjoy white flour baking just occasionally, which is the perfect balance for me. Make this delicate loaf when you want to fill the kitchen with the aroma of herbs. It's also a satisfying bread for new or young cooks to try. Try it spread with a little Mung Bean Pâté (page 77), or sliced thinly, toasted, and served with Alphabet Soup (page 95).

MAKES 2 LOAVES

PREPARATION TIME 1¼ HOURS

1 heaped teaspoon sugar

1 × 8g sachet or 2 teaspoons dried yeast

500g (1lb 2oz/3⅓ cups) strong white flour

3 tablespoons extra virgin olive oil, plus extra for oiling the baking sheets and your hands

2 tablespoons dried rosemary

1 tablespoon dried sage

OPTIONS AND VARIATIONS

Use a cooking brush to lightly oil the top of the freshly baked loaves and immediately sprinkle a little coarse salt onto the oiled surface.

Measure 250ml (9fl oz/1 cup) warm (blood temperature) water into a measuring jug (large measuring cup), and dissolve the sugar in it. Add the yeast, stir well and set the mixture aside to turn frothy.

Measure the flour into a large bowl, and make a well in the centre.

When the yeast mixture is frothy, stir in the oil and then pour the yeast and oil mixture into the flour. Measure another 100ml (3½fl oz/ scant ½ cup) warm water into the jug, and keep it near to hand.

Stir together the flour and liquid with a wooden spoon until it becomes difficult. Scrape the dough from the spoon and begin to knead the dough with your hands, adding a little of the extra water if needed. Aim to make a firm dough that is not sticky. Cover the bowl with a clean tea towel, and leave the dough to rise for 30 minutes

Meanwhile, crush the dried herbs using a mortar and pestle, or in a bowl with a wooden spoon. When the dough has risen, tip the herbs over the dough. Lightly oil two baking sheets, and rub a little of this oil onto your hands as you begin to knead the herbs into the dough.

Divide the dough in two. Lift one half to eye level and, using both hands, swiftly elongate it to form a thick rope. Immediately fold the rope in half and twist the two halves against each other. The twist should be 25–30cm (10–12in) long. Immediately rest it onto one of the baking sheets, then repeat this manoeuvre for the second portion of dough.

Cover the loaves with a tea towel, and set aside to rise for 30 minutes.

Preheat the oven to 200°C (400°F). Bake the loaves in the hot oven for 5 minutes, then reduce the temperature to 180°C (350°F) and bake for a further 20–25 minutes. Allow the loaves to cool on their baking sheets for 5 minutes, before transferring to a wire rack to cool.

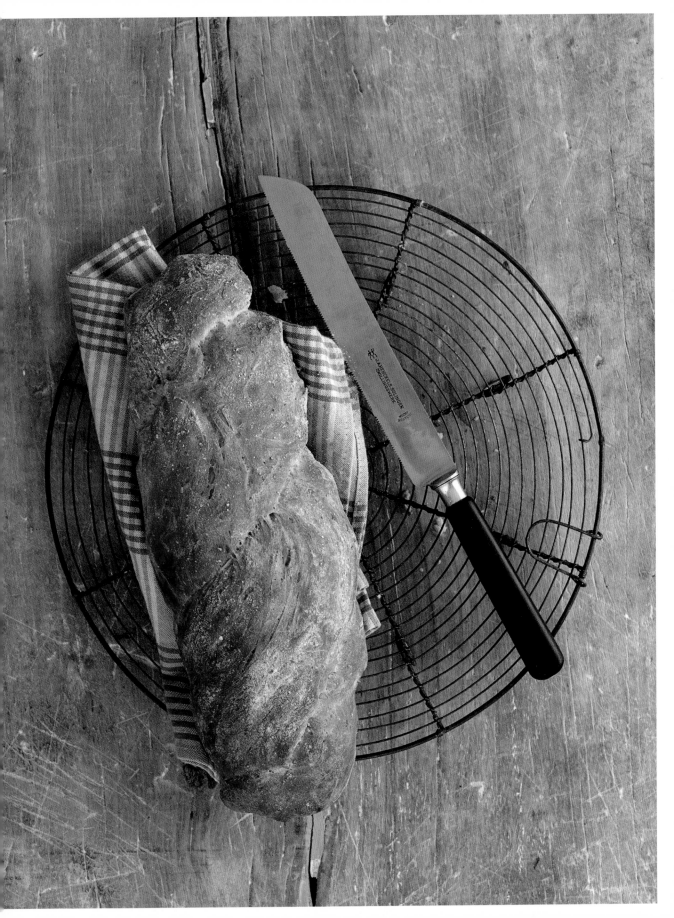

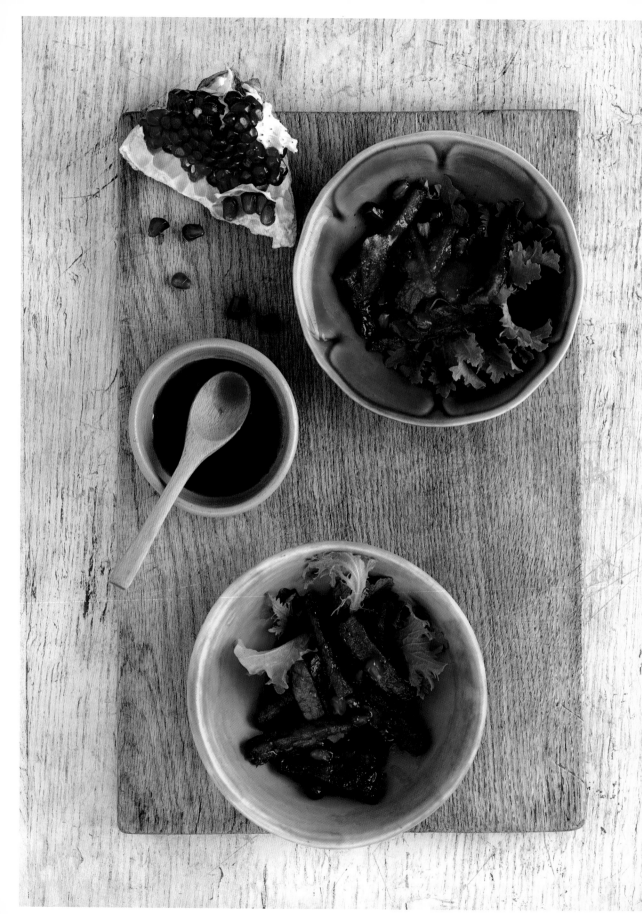

TEMPEH CRISPS IN POMEGRANATE GLAZE

This simple delicacy holds that special place on the plate reserved for high-protein dishes. I always make double quantities because the tempeh crisps are very easy to eat. Excellent as a starter (appetizer) or beside Sautéed Tatsoi in Black Sesame (page 112) and Yellow Rice Zinger (page 129).

SERVES 4

PREPARATION TIME 40 MINUTES

400g (14oz) tempeh

3 tablespoons untoasted sesame oil

Juice of 2 limes

1 tablespoon tamari

3 tablespoons pomegranate molasses

OPTIONS AND VARIATIONS

Add a pinch of black pepper to the glaze mixture.

Slice the tempeh into thin strips about 1cm (½in) thick) of any shape.

Pour half the oil into a frying pan (skillet) and arrange the tempeh slices in it. Set the pan over a medium heat and begin to sauté the tempeh, moving the slices now and then so that they don't stick. Turn the slices so that both sides become brown and crisp, adding more of the oil if needed. I generally allow 10–12 minutes' cooking time on each side.

Meanwhile, prepare the glaze: in a measuring jug (large measuring cup) or small bowl, stir together the lime juice, tamari and 2 tablespoons of the pomegranate molasses.

Arrange the cooked tempeh on a shallow serving dish.

Pour the glaze mixture into the hot pan, stir it around for a minute to gather any residual oils and flavours, then pour it over the tempeh.

Drizzle the remaining 1 tablespoon molasses in a crisscross pattern over the tempeh. Serve immediately.

✳ **TEMPEH** is made from soya beans and so is very high in protein. Soya can sometimes be hard for people to digest, but as tempeh is fermented it is actually very easy to digest. During one of my pregnancies, I ate tempeh every day for the first three months. In fact, I craved it. I found it light and comfortable to eat, and it certainly did its work: he was a nine-pound baby.

TEMPEH, LETTUCE AND TOMATO SANDWICH (TLT)

Make a simple, bold challenge to the famous but outdated BLT with this wholesome sandwich. Tempeh is inexpensive, quick to prepare, and richly nutritious. Develop the theme by spreading 2 tablespoons Herb and Onion Bean Butter (page 71) onto the bread instead of the olive oil, or adding a dollop of Tofu-Mayo (page 99) or a sprinkling of Sprouted Mung Beans (page 78). Bet you can't make just one!

MAKES 1 SANDWICH

PREPARATION TIME 20 MINUTES

1 tablespoon untoasted sesame oil

100g (3½oz) tempeh, cut into slices no more than 1cm (½in) thick

2 slices of favourite bread

1 teaspoon extra virgin olive oil

1 teaspoon favourite mustard

2 lettuce leaves

1 tomato, sliced

Dash of tamari and/or hot sauce

OPTIONS AND VARIATIONS

You know how to make your own sandwich: swap the order in which you layer the ingredients, add more or less of what you like, add other sauces, and so on. Toss some thinly sliced onion in the hot pan for a moment, and add to the layers.

Heat the oil in a frying pan (skillet) set over a medium heat. Add the tempeh slices to the pan and cook for about 7 minutes on each side, until they are golden brown, aromatic and with a hint of crispiness.

Meanwhile, toast the bread. Drizzle both pieces of toast with olive oil and then spread a thin layer of mustard onto each slice.

Arrange the lettuce and tomato on one of the slices, and top with the cooked tempeh. Sprinkle a little tamari and/or hot sauce onto the hot tempeh.

Close the sandwich and serve hot.

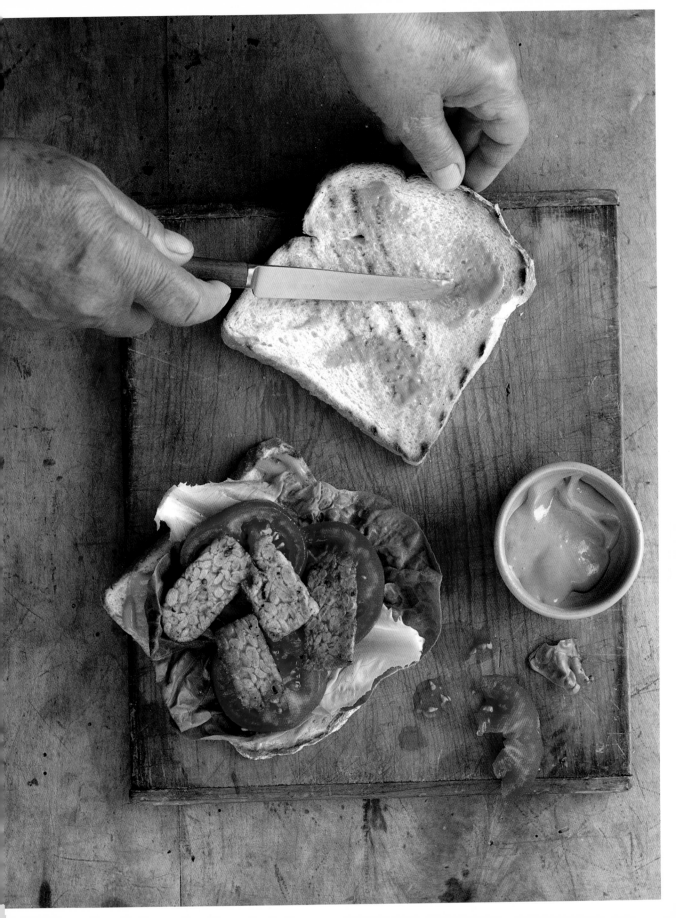

SORREL SOUP

Surprising, tangy flavours emerge from this tender leaf. Some call it a bitter leaf, others sour; it has a definite lemon tone. I find it very more-ish, whether in soup or salad, and am always sorry when its season ends, toward the end of summer. I like this soup served hot, but not too hot, with a slice of Eat-It-Today Cornbread (page 135).

SERVES 4

PREPARATION TIME 30 MINUTES

1 tablespoon untoasted sesame oil

1 medium white potato, cubed

1 medium onion, finely chopped

1 small leek, finely chopped

1 teaspoon vegan bouillon powder

¼ teaspoon black pepper

125g (4½oz) fresh sorrel, chopped

OPTIONS AND VARIATIONS

Add up to 200g (7oz) fresh sorrel to this soup – an extra 75g (2½oz) – if desired. The leaves reduce significantly in volume when cooked.

Pour the oil into a saucepan set over a medium heat. Add the potato, onion and leek. Cover the pan and sauté for 15 minutes, stirring twice in that time.

Stir in the bouillon powder and black pepper. When the onion and leek are tender, add the sorrel and cook for a further 3–5 minutes.

Spoon about one-third of this mixture into a bowl and set aside.

Add 1 litre (35fl oz/4 cups) water to the mixture remaining in the pan, and purée using a hand-held blender. Cover the pan and bring to a low simmer.

Return the reserved sorrel mixture to the pan. Stir well and remove from the heat. Serve hot.

CHOC HOTLATE

There are times when a cup of chocolatey warmth is the only thing that matters. Maybe chocolate really is a health food!

MAKES 1 MUGFUL

PREPARATION TIME 10 MINUTES

250ml (9fl oz/1 cup) plant milk

1 teaspoon barley malt syrup

1 teaspoon unsweetened, dairy-free cocoa powder

1 small square (about 5g) from a bar of 70% dark chocolate

1 tablespoon of rice or soya ice cream

OPTIONS AND VARIATIONS

Sprinkle a tiny pinch of cayenne pepper over the grated chocolate, before the ice cream.

Warm the milk, syrup and cocoa in a small saucepan over a low heat, stirring or whisking to ensure an even distribution. When it seems about to simmer, remove the pan from the heat and pour its contents into a mug.

Grate a little chocolate from the bar onto the hot milk, and top with the ice cream. Serve immediately, with a spoon.

✳ **DARK CHOCOLATE** is very rich in magnesium, iron and zinc, and is abundant in plant chemicals, called flavanols, that are thought to have a protective effect on the heart. Buying 70% dark chocolate (or higher) will provide useful amounts of the beneficial nutrients as well as the slightly bitter taste that is a signature of good chocolate. Interestingly, you probably won't crave more and more of dark chocolate; it is lower in sugar than milk chocolate and creates satiety, a sense of 'that's enough.' I was once given a great gift: a kit for making dark chocolate. I really appreciated using the organic, Fair Trade ingredients and seeing, for the first time ever, what goes into making a piece of chocolate. As a result of that experience, I now purchase dark chocolate made by artisans who use ingredients from growers' cooperatives. It is very easy to find these products now and, in my opinion, they put dark chocolate into the category of a really classy treat.

GRILLED ORANGES WITH MAPLE SYRUP

Intense flavours are the signature of this simple dessert. Serve hot or cold, but always on your prettiest plates, and provide a sharp knife, fork and spoon. To eat, begin by pulling away the pointy tips of peel at the ends of each quarter – this should happen quite easily once started. Then use the knife and fork to cut bite-sized pieces of orange away from the peel, and dip each piece of orange into the little mound of nuts and syrup. There is a messier way to eat these: simply pick up one of the quarters, holding onto the two pointy tips. Bring it close to your mouth and bite into the orange. It will pull neatly away from the peel with only a drip or two to tidy up. Enjoy the little bits of charred pith, too.

SERVES 4

PREPARATION TIME 20 MINUTES

4 large oranges, quartered
from top to bottom

4 tablespoons crushed walnuts

4 tablespoons maple syrup

OPTIONS AND VARIATIONS

Use crushed hazelnuts instead
of the walnuts.

Preheat the grill (broiler) until hot. Arrange the orange quarters resting on their peel on a baking sheet, with the core of the orange facing upwards.

Grill (broil) the oranges for 10–12 minutes, turning the baking sheet once in that time. Let the oranges cool for 5 minutes, then arrange on individual serving plates.

Put a portion of the crushed walnuts on one side of each plate, pour a little syrup over the nuts, and serve.

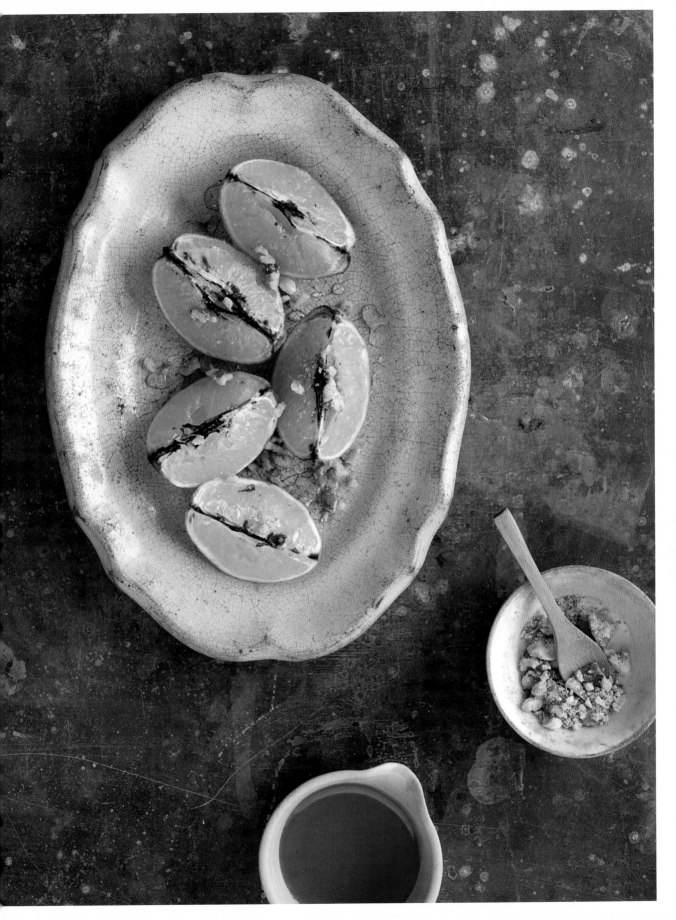

FAMILY DINNERS

ROAST DINNER MEDLEY

I love how this meal can help people to relax and sit a bit longer in conversation. The autumn (fall) colours are celebrated in its selection of roots: maple-leaf purple, orange, white, palest yellow and darkest red. Pack the oven full of roasting dishes, use the stovetop to cook something green – steam 500g (1lb 2 oz) Brussels sprouts or boil the same amount of green peas – and then call everyone to the table. Top the whole lot with Gravy of the Gods (page 208) and serve with a Quick Patty Cake Mix version of a vegan roast (page 50).

SERVES 4

PREPARATION TIME 1¼ HOURS

Oil for greasing the baking dishes

500g (1lb 2oz) Vitelotte purple potatoes

500g (1lb 2 oz) La Ratte potatoes

4 small beetroot (beets)

4 medium parsnips, quartered along their length

4 medium carrots, quartered along their length

4 small turnips, quartered

OPTIONS AND VARIATIONS

If your oven can take it, quarter and deseed a small pumpkin and roast for 25 minutes, uncovered, with a little water in the bottom of the roasting pan. Or you could steam the pumpkin quarters on the stovetop.

Preheat the oven to 200°C (400°F) and lightly oil two baking dishes: a large one for the potatoes and a medium one for the parsnips, carrots and turnips. (You'll also need a small to medium covered dish for baking the beetroot – but you do not oil this dish.)

Cut the potatoes into 6cm (2½in) chunks and put them in the large dish. Jostle them to get a coating of oil over them. Put the dish on the top shelf of the oven.

Add water to a depth of 3cm (1¼in) to the covered baking dish. Place the beetroot upside down, so that they are standing on their trimmed stalks in the water, and cover the dish. Put in the oven on the shelf below the potatoes.

Mix the parsnips, carrots and turnip in their baking dish, jostling them to coat with oil. Put this dish in the oven about 10 minutes after the potatoes and beetroot, on the shelf next to the beetroot. (You're aiming for everything to be ready at the same time – the potatoes and beetroot need to cook for about 40 minutes, the parsnips and carrots about 30).

ALMOND, LIME AND FRESH HERB PESTO

You could use a blender here – but I find it takes longer to clean the machine afterwards than it does to make the pesto by hand! In any case, I always enjoy the scent of the herbs as I prepare them. Try making this with various aromatic leaves. My favourite combinations include: lemon balm and mint; wild garlic (ramps), land cress and parsley; rocket (arugula) and sorrel; or mustard and shiso leaves. Stir a heaped tablespoon of pesto into a bowl of pasta, dollop onto a baked potato, or spread a little onto freshly baked Rosemary Twist (page 164).

MAKES ABOUT 250ML (1 CUP)

PREPARATION TIME 15 MINUTES

100g (3½oz) fresh herbs, leaves picked over and stems discarded

25g (1oz/¼ cup) ground almonds

¼ teaspoon black pepper

Pinch of salt

Juice of 2 limes

120ml (4fl oz/½ cup) extra virgin olive oil, plus a little extra for covering the pesto in the jar

OPTIONS AND VARIATIONS

For a spicier pesto, replace the black pepper with cayenne pepper.

Press the herbs together in a firm mound on a board. Chop them as finely as you can, then put them in a small mixing bowl.

Stir in the ground almonds, black pepper, salt, lime juice and olive oil. Using a wooden spoon, stir the mixture for 1–2 minutes to ensure the almonds are evenly distributed. Pack the pesto into a clean jar.

Level the pesto and pour over sufficient olive oil to thinly cover the surface. Put the lid on the jar and refrigerate until ready to use. If you can, leave the pesto to stand for at least 4 hours before you eat it, to allow the flavours to mature.

The pesto will keep for 3–4 days if you ensure that it is covered with a little olive oil before returning it to the refrigerator.

✳ **OLIVE OIL** has been used for thousands of years: as a lamp oil, as an emollient for the skin, as a medicine and as a cornerstone of what is now called the 'Mediterranean diet'. It is the food oil highest in monounsaturated fatty acids. It can help to prevent the build-up of 'bad' cholesterol and does not reduce the level of 'good' cholesterol in the blood.

✳ **WHEN BUYING OLIVE OIL** select extra virgin olive oil that is cold-pressed and unrefined. It will have a strong flavour and a greenish colour. It is worth the extra cost. Do not cook with extra virgin olive oil (heat will destroy much of its health-giving properties), but use it freely in dressings, dips, spreads or, as in this recipe, as a gentle, flavoursome aid to preservation. Beware of olive oil labelled 'pure', as it has probably been refined and its nutrient value reduced as a result.

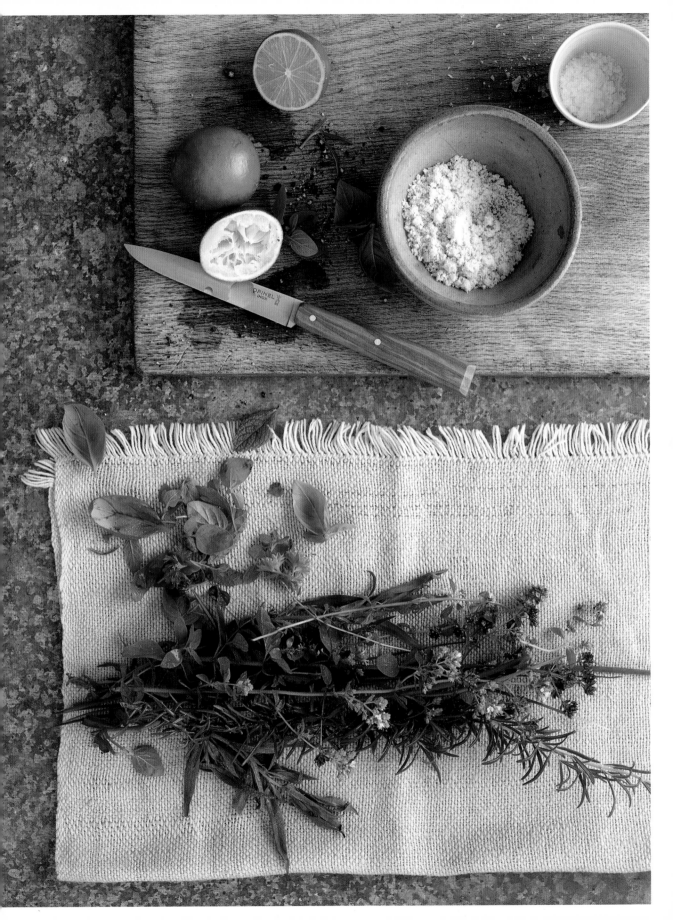

WHITE SAUCE BASICS

My great-grandmother taught me how to make a white sauce. She also showed me how to bottle fresh peaches, how to make doughnuts, and how to dress the burn I got from splashing the hot oil. I am grateful that she shared so much of what she knew. Here is the simple idea behind the sauce. You need only to try it once, after which you will know the technique and be able to use it to create soups and sauces. It starts by making an oil and water paste, which the French call a *roux*; it will thicken any liquid you add to it. The paste also will act as a vehicle for herbs, spices and all manner of flavours.

MAKES 1 LITRE (4 CUPS)

PREPARATION TIME 15 MINUTES

70ml (2¼fl oz) untoasted sesame oil

70g (2½oz/½ cup) plain (all-purpose) flour

1 litre (35fl oz/4 cups) plant milk or Homemade Vegetable Stock (page 185), or a combination of both

OPTIONS AND VARIATIONS

Dried herbs and spices can be added to the flour, while chopped fresh herbs should be added after the sauce is completed, cooking them briefly to release their flavour. Add finely chopped vegetables, such as mushrooms, garlic, onions or sweet pepper (capsicum) to the oil and sauté them until tender, before adding the flour. Although the basic recipe is for a 'white' sauce, you can add ingredients to change its colour. Ground turmeric will turn the sauce yellow and also further thicken it. Mustard powder will do the same – it is hotter than prepared mustard, but you can also try prepared Dijon or wholegrain mustards.

Heat the oil in a saucepan over a low heat. Sprinkle in the flour and stir with a wooden spoon. As the flour cooks, it will absorb the oil and form a thick paste.

(You can remove the pan from the heat at this point, until you are ready to complete your sauce. You can even store the cooked flour and oil paste for a short time in the refrigerator and warm it when you are ready to use it. If you want to do this, you'll get a smoother sauce if you bring the milk or stock to a simmer in a separate pan before adding it to the reheated paste, as in the following instructions.)

Add milk or stock a little at a time to the flour and oil paste, stirring all the while over the heat. The paste will disperse and the liquid will thicken. Keep stirring and adding liquid until the sauce is the thickness you desire. Cook for about 2 minutes, then remove from the heat.

ABSOLUTELY GREEN SAUCE This sauce makes a simple but pleasing topping to a baked potato or a bowl of naked pasta. It brings together two strong-minded herbs: parsley, for its down-to-earth green flavour, and watercress, for its pepperiness. Different plant milks will give varied results: soya milk will allow the herb flavours to come to the fore, while coconut or almond milks will impart their own flavours. Decide which milk works best for you (or leave out the milk completely and use only vegetable stock). To make about 500ml (17fl oz/2 cups), heat 1 tablespoon untoasted sesame oil in a saucepan and sprinkle 1 tablespoon plain (all-purpose) flour and a pinch each of black pepper and nutmeg over the hot oil. Stir well to create a thick paste. Measure 500ml (17fl oz/2 cups) plant milk or vegetable stock, or 250ml (9fl oz/1 cup) of each, and gradually add this liquid to the paste. Stir well after each addition to create a smooth sauce. Add 10g (¼oz/⅓ cup) finely chopped flat-leaf parsley and 10g (¼oz/⅓ cup) finely chopped watercress, stir well and continue to cook for a further 5 minutes. Serve hot.

SEARED VEGETABLES WITH LEMON TARRAGON SAUCE

Make the sauce first because the vegetables are very quick to cook. This delicate, creamy sauce is perfect for summer dishes. Pick tarragon fresh from its stalk from mid June through to the end of August; it adds an aromatic, slightly anise-flavoured tone to this sauce. Pour a little over new potatoes or Polenta with Garden Garland (page 100). It combines rather well with Seaweed and Potato Cutlets (page 206), too.

SERVES 4

PREPARATION TIME 30 MINUTES

Juice of 2 lemons

Grated zest of 1 lemon

2 tablespoons finely chopped fresh tarragon

2 tablespoons untoasted sesame oil

1 tablespoon plain (all-purpose) flour

200ml (7fl oz/scant 1 cup) almond milk

10g (¼oz) dried arame

1 tender leek, cut into thin coins

¼ head of small white cabbage, shredded

½ teaspoon black pepper

OPTIONS AND VARIATIONS

Use cashew or hazelnut milk instead of almond milk. Garnish with chopped tarragon or a few shreds of grated lemon zest.

Stir together the lemon juice, lemon zest and tarragon in a bowl or measuring jug (large measuring cup), and set to one side.

Heat 1 tablespoon of the oil in a small saucepan over a medium heat. Sprinkle in the flour, stirring as it thickens to a paste, about 5 minutes. Gradually add the almond milk, a little at a time, stirring constantly to create a smooth sauce.

Slowly add the lemon and herb mixture, stirring constantly. Remove from the heat and tip the sauce into a jug (pitcher). Keep warm.

Meanwhile, soak the arame in a bowl of cold water. Heat the remaining tablespoon of oil in a large frying pan (skillet) over a medium-high heat. Add the leek and cabbage, and stir them together in the pan. Cover the pan and cook for 5 minutes.

Drain and rinse the arame and add to the pan. Add the black pepper, stir the vegetables and leave them to cook, covered, for a further 5 minutes over a medium heat. Serve hot with the warm Lemon Tarragon Sauce.

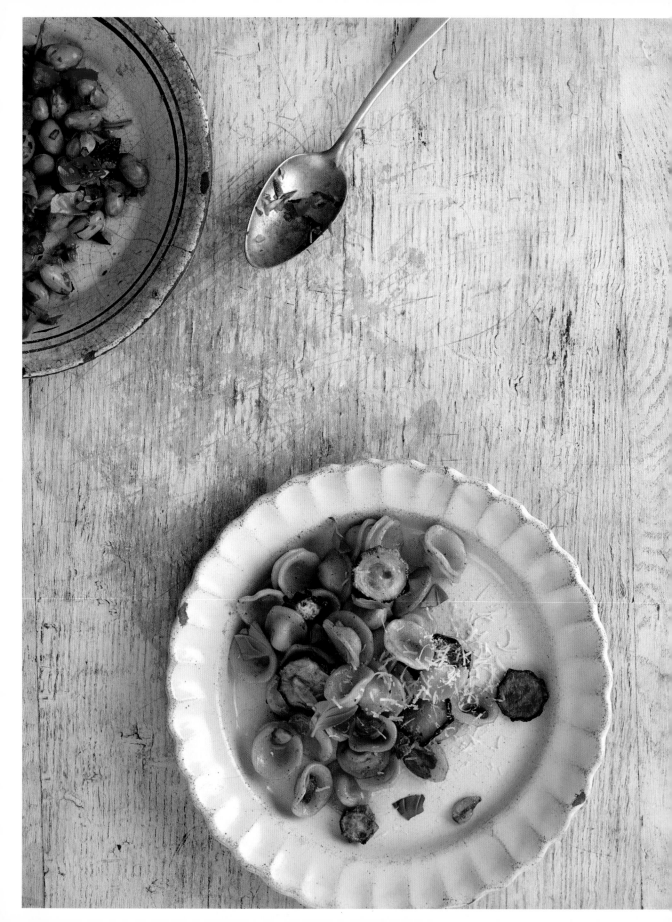

ORECCHIETTE WITH GARLIC, BASIL AND TOASTED COURGETTE

Orecchiette, meaning 'little ears', is a type of pasta that is popular in the Puglia region of Italy. It is traditionally made by hand – the thumb pressing its shape into a pinch of dough – and I have watched the local women making it as they stand chatting together in their sunny courtyards. Each little ear is then dropped onto a wire mesh rack and left to dry in the open air. This dish is quick and simple to make, and Fresh Borlotti Bean Salad (page 104) is an excellent side.

Preheat the grill (broiler) until hot, and set a large pot of water to come to a boil for the pasta.

Arrange the courgette coins in a single layer on a baking sheet, and cook under the hot grill for 1 minute. Use a spatula to turn them and grill for a further 1 minute. The slices will swell slightly and develop a lightly coloured, toasted surface that helps them to retain their shape.

Pour the oil into a large frying pan (skillet) set over a medium heat. Add the garlic, spices and toasted courgette slices. Cover the pan and sauté for about 5 minutes until the garlic is just tender.

Add the orecchiette to the boiling water and cook according to the packet instructions (usually 8–10 minutes), stirring frequently, until just tender.

Drain the pasta and stir some of the garlic and courgette mixture into each portion. Sprinkle fresh basil over each plate and serve.

SERVES 4

PREPARATION TIME 35 MINUTES

3 medium courgettes (zucchini), sliced into coins

1 tablespoon untoasted sesame oil

1 whole garlic bulb, cloves separated and sliced

½ teaspoon ground cinnamon

¼ teaspoon black pepper

500g (1lb 2oz) dried orecchiette

4 large sprigs of fresh basil, chopped

OPTIONS AND VARIATIONS

Grate a little Mozzarella-type vegan cheese or Parmesan-type vegan cheese (often sold as 'vegan grating cheese') over each serving.

PENNE WITH SEASONAL GREENS

I always feel a burst of energy after making this dish. Fresh greens are highly nutritious and this dish delivers their nutrients in glorious abundance. I match this dish to the seasons by using whatever greens are fresh and new to the market stalls.

SERVES 4

PREPARATION TIME 45 MINUTES

2 tablespoons untoasted sesame oil

4 litres (140fl oz/16 cups) chopped mixed seasonal greens, such as cavolo nero, tatsoi, mustard greens, dandelion leaves, Tenderstem or purple sprouting broccoli, small amounts of spinach, rocket (arugula) and chicory

1 tablespoon dried basil

1 teaspoon dried oregano

1 fresh chilli, finely chopped, or ½ teaspoon chilli flakes

¼ teaspoon ground nutmeg

1 whole garlic bulb, cloves separated and chopped

500g (1lb 2oz) dried penne

Extra virgin olive oil for drizzling

OPTIONS AND VARIATIONS

Add a handful of cherry tomatoes to the cooking greens – they will burst and add colour. You could try other short pasta shapes.

Pour the oil into a large (4-litre/140fl oz/16-cup) saucepan. If you don't have a 4-litre pan, use the largest one you have and fill it with greens. Press and pack the chopped greens into the pan. It should be absolutely full!

Cover the pan and place over a medium-high heat for 5 minutes.

If you have used a smaller pan, add the remaining greens and the herbs, spices and garlic. There will be room – the greens will reduce in bulk very quickly. Reduce the heat to medium and cook for 12–15 minutes, stirring occasionally.

Meanwhile, bring a large pot of water to the boil. Add the penne and cook according to the packet instructions until just tender. Drain the pasta into a colander and return it to the hot pan. Stir the greens through the pasta and serve, drizzling a little extra virgin olive oil over each serving.

✳ **GREEN JUICES** You will notice that some greens produce more juices than others when they are cooked. This is normal and depends on how fresh the greens are as well as what specific plant is used. Cos (romaine) lettuce and pak choi (bok choy), for instance, release more juices than broccoli or white cabbage; but all greens release some. You can make adjustments to the amount of liquid by adding 1–2 tablespoons water or sauce, if needed; or, as in the options, by adding a few cherry tomatoes.

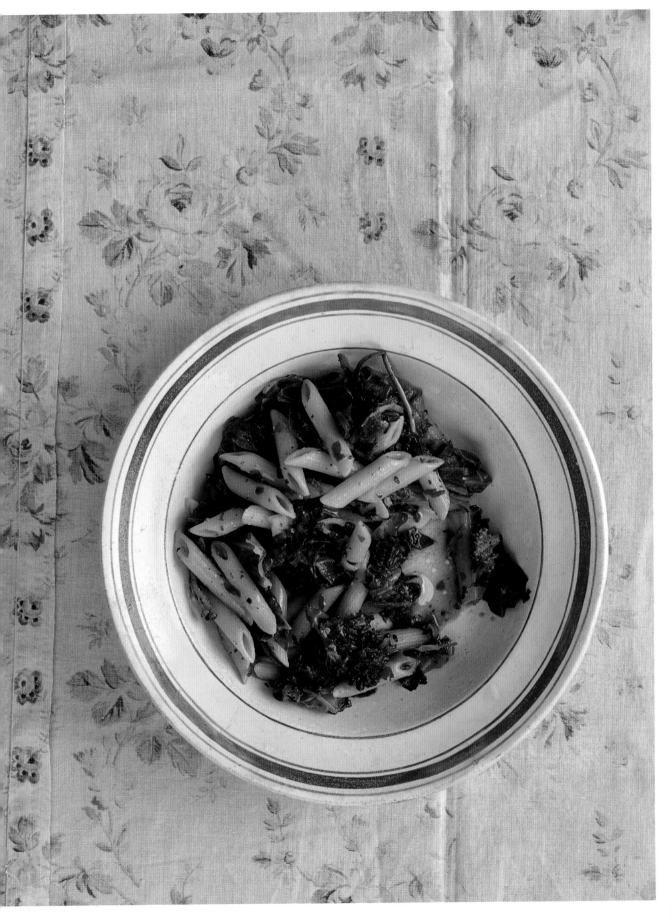

THREE-GRAIN RISOTTO

This combination of wholesome grains with aromatic herbs and spices looks splendid, and makes a substantial side dish or a bed for vegetables or beans. Wild rice has a unique aroma and texture, as well as a distinctive black colour. For a neat presentation, press portions of risotto into small, slightly dampened bowls, wait a moment, then turn the bowls upside down onto a plate to give a perfectly formed dome of rice. Serve with Sautéed Tatsoi in Black Sesame (page 112) and Carrot, Arame and Ginger Sauté (page 195); or with Chunky Tofu in Greens (page 117).

SERVES 4

PREPARATION TIME 1 HOUR

2 tablespoons untoasted sesame oil

1 medium onion, finely chopped

10g (¼oz/⅓ cup) chopped fresh flat-leaf parsley

1 teaspoon dried basil

½ teaspoon dried oregano

¼ teaspoon ground cinnamon

¼ teaspoon black pepper

100g (3½oz/½ cup) wild rice

100g (3½oz/½ cup) short-grain brown rice

50g (1¾oz) millet

500ml (17fl oz/2 cups) vegetable stock

OPTIONS AND VARIATIONS

Add 4 chopped garlic cloves with the herbs and spices. Wild rice can sometimes be hard to find – if so, use red or black rice instead. If you run out of vegetable stock, use boiling water as needed.

Heat the oil in a large saucepan, and sauté the onion for 10 minutes over a low heat until softened.

Meanwhile, put the stock in a separate pan and bring to a simmer.

Add the herbs and spices to the onion, stir well and sauté for about 2 more minutes. Increase the heat to medium.

Mix together the two rices in a bowl, cover with water and stir them around to wash. Drain well, then add the grain mixture to the pan and stir until the oil has been absorbed. Pour in 100ml (3½fl oz/scant ½ cup) of the hot stock and stir until absorbed.

Add more stock until it just covers the grain mixture. Cover the pan and let its contents cook over a low to medium heat. After 15 minutes, check to see whether the grain has absorbed the stock. Stir gently to check the texture of the grains; they should be swollen but not quite tender. Add 100ml (3½fl oz/scant ½ cup) stock or water, cover the pan and continue cooking over a low heat for a further 15 minutes or so. Check the grains during this time, adding more liquid if needed, and cook until the grains are tender and the liquid fully absorbed.

HOMEMADE VEGETABLE STOCK

I tend to have vegan bouillon powder in the cupboard somewhere, but I find it very satisfying to make my own stock and usually prepare it while cooking other dishes. I use the ragged trimmings from fresh vegetables, such as the tough ends of celery stalks, frayed tips of greens, outer leaves of cabbage and even a sprig or two of green carrot top. It's a great way to collect flavours and nutrients that might otherwise have been discarded (just ensure that whatever you add is properly washed). When the stock is cool, I strain it, pour it into containers (including ice-cube trays) and freeze. It comes in very handy; I use it instead of water to make soups or sauces, to cook rice or even in making bread.

MAKES 1¼ LITRES (6 CUPS)

PREPARATION TIME 45 MINUTES

2 tablespoons untoasted sesame oil

1 large onion, chopped

2 celery stalks, chopped

1 medium carrot, chopped

1 medium potato, chopped

1 medium turnip, chopped

Green trimmings from cauliflower, broccoli or cabbage, cleaned and chopped

10cm (4in) strip of kombu, rinsed

2 bay leaves

2 sage leaves, fresh or dried

50g (1¾oz/about 1½ cups) coarsely chopped fresh flat-leaf parsley (including stalks)

1 teaspoon dried basil

½ teaspoon dried marjoram or oregano

¼ teaspoon black pepper

¼ teaspoon ground nutmeg

Pour the oil into a large stockpot or saucepan set over a medium heat. Add the onion and vegetables to the pan, and cook, covered, for 10 minutes.

Add the kombu, herbs and spices, and cook a further 5 minutes. Pour in 2 litres (70fl oz/8 cups) water, stir well and increase the heat to bring the water to a boil. Reduce the heat and simmer the broth for 30 minutes, covered, without disturbing.

Remove from the heat and strain the stock for immediate use. If you plan to use the stock later, leave to cool before straining.

SAUTÉED JERUSALEM ARTICHOKES AND SWEET POTATOES

Jerusalem artichokes are tubers from the sunflower family of plants. They cook in about the same time as sweet potato, and the two make a great pair in colour, texture and flavour. Both of them give this dish a lovely caramelized surface. Serve with Sweetcorn and Pepper Relish (page 134), a portion of Dressed Greens and Beans (page 154) and perhaps a slice of Eat-It-Today Cornbread (page 135).

SERVES 4

PREPARATION TIME 30 MINUTES

1 tablespoon untoasted sesame oil

300g (10½oz) Jerusalem artichokes, sliced into 1cm (½in) thick rounds

1 medium sweet potato, cut into chunks

2 spring onions (scallions), finely chopped

3 tablespoons chopped fresh flat-leaf parsley

¼ teaspoon Chinese five-spice

¼ teaspoon black pepper

Zest and juice of 1 lemon

1 tablespoon tamari

OPTIONS AND VARIATIONS

Add 6 chopped garlic cloves, right at the start of cooking the roots.

Heat the oil in a large frying pan (skillet) set over a medium heat. Add the sliced artichoke and sweet potato. Cover the pan and sauté, turning now and then so they are evenly cooked, for about 20 minutes.

Meanwhile, in a bowl, mix together the spring onions, parsley, spices, lemon zest and juice.

When the artichokes and sweet potato are tender, transfer them to a serving dish.

Pour the spring onion mixture into the hot frying pan. Stir and cover the pan, then cook for 3 minutes.

Remove the pan from the heat and add the tamari. Stir well and tip this mixture over the artichokes and sweet potatoes.

Serve immediately.

✱ **JERUSALEM ARTICHOKES** can sometimes be quite small and I find it is best to use these first, as they can simply shrivel if left too long. The little ones can be difficult to hold on to when I try to scrub them, so I have taken to soaking them in cold water first, just for 5 minutes. This loosens the dirt and makes the scrubbing easier. No matter what size they are, after a good scrubbing I always soak them for a further 5 minutes to remove any possibility of grittiness.

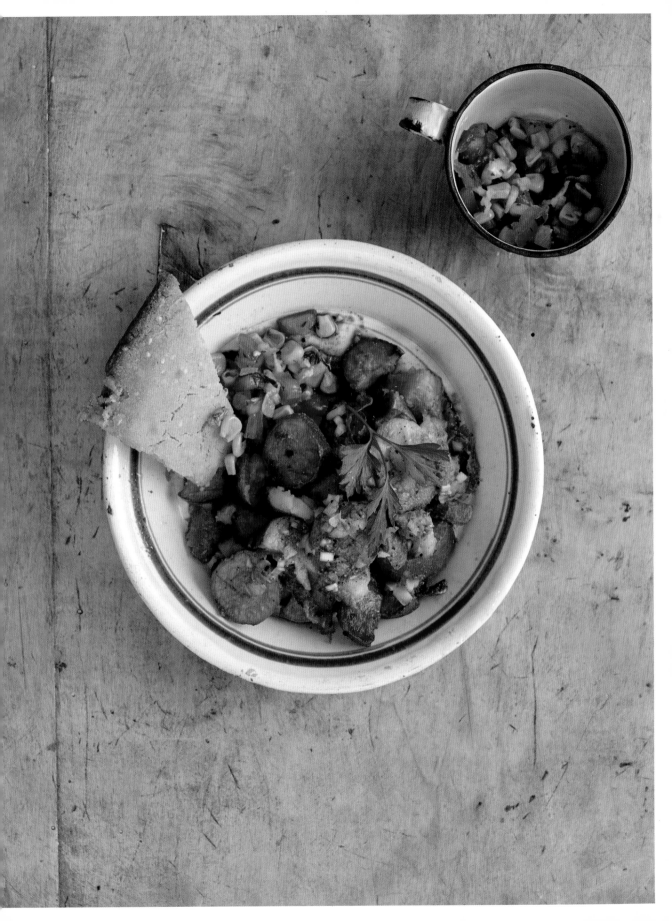

BAKED BOUNTIFUL

Put this together before work, set the timer on your oven and come home to a hot, aromatic meal. It is really very quick to set up. Delicious with peas or a serving of Precious Greens (page 193).

SERVES 4

PREPARATION TIME 1 HOUR

1 tablespoon untoasted sesame oil

4 medium potatoes, sliced

2 medium carrots, sliced

2 medium onions, chopped

200g (7oz) coarsely chopped greens, such as spinach, cavolo nero or pak choi (bok choy)

2 tablespoons vegan gravy powder

1 teaspoon dried basil

1 teaspoon dried oregano

½ teaspoon black pepper

OPTIONS AND VARIATIONS

Use slices of sweet potato instead of the top layer of potato. If your ovenproof dish can take it, add extra layers of different vegetables, such as sliced parsnips – and then add a little more gravy.

Preheat the oven to 200°C (400°F), and brush the oil over the inside of a 3-litre (100fl oz/12-cup) ovenproof dish (one that has a lid).

Arrange half of the potatoes in a layer covering the bottom of the dish. Layer all the carrots over the potatoes. Ensure that the layers extend evenly to the edges of the dish, and that you don't end up with a mound in the middle. Cut some of the slices of potato or carrot in half, if needed. Spread half of the chopped onions over the carrots, then layer all of the greens on top, pressing them firmly in place. Arrange the remaining onions over the greens, and top with the remaining potatoes.

In a jug (large measuring cup), mix together the gravy powder, basil, oregano and black pepper. Add a little cold water to make a smooth paste. Add 750ml (26fl oz/3 cups) cold water to the paste and stir well. Pour the gravy mixture over the layered vegetables.

Cover the dish and bake in the oven for 45–60 minutes until the vegetables are tender. Serve in great spoonfuls, making sure to slice down through all the layers.

SCALLOPED POTATO BAKE

Perhaps your grandmother made something similar to this simple dish – it goes with almost anything. It's substantial and warming, and is a good recipe for young people to learn. Try it served with Precious Greens (page 193) and Chickpea and Ruby Chard Hubbub (page 198).

SERVES 4

PREPARATION TIME 1 HOUR

500g (1lb 2 oz) potatoes

1 medium onion, finely chopped

60g (2¼oz/scant ½ cup) plain (all-purpose) flour

½ teaspoon black pepper

½ teaspoon caraway seeds, crushed

Pinch of salt

Oil for drizzling

400ml (14fl oz) plant milk

50g (1¾oz/½ cup) dried breadcrumbs

OPTIONS AND VARIATIONS

Use ½ teaspoon mustard powder instead of the black pepper. Sprinkle 1 teaspoon nutritional yeast flakes between each layer of potato. Use tiny dollops of vegan margarine, instead of the oil, between layers. Crush plain water biscuits (crackers) over the top layer instead of the breadcrumbs.

Preheat the oven to 200°C (400°F), and oil a 1-litre (35fl oz/4-cup) baking dish.

Slice the potatoes into thin rounds, no more than 1cm (½in) thick, and arrange a layer in the bottom of the baking dish. Sprinkle some of the chopped onion over the potato layer.

Mix together the flour, pepper and caraway seeds in a small bowl. Sprinkle a little of this mixture over the onion, then scatter over a pinch of salt. Drizzle 1 tablespoon oil over the flour mixture.

Repeat the layers, ending with a layer of potato. Pour over the plant milk and sprinkle the breadcrumbs over the top.

Pop the dish in the oven, and bake for 45–50 minutes until the potatoes are tender. Serve hot.

BROCCOLI ALMOND SIZZLE

I love this simple and pretty dish. It offers interesting taste and texture surprises to complement the strong green flavour of the broccoli. I like to have it with a bowl of noodles or serve it as one of three or four dishes to make a hearty dinner. Serve it with Jerusalem Artichoke and Sweet Potato Sauté (page 186) or Scalloped Potato Bake (page 189).

SERVES 4

PREPARATION TIME 20 MINUTES

1 tablespoon untoasted sesame oil

1 head of broccoli, florets halved or quartered

1 red onion, halved and thinly sliced

50g (1¾oz/½ cup) flaked almonds

¼ teaspoon black pepper

¼ teaspoon ground allspice

Juice of 1 lime

OPTIONS AND VARIATIONS

Stems of purple sprouting broccoli or florets of cauliflower may be mixed, half and half, with the regular broccoli to create a multicoloured dish.

Pour the oil into a large frying pan (skillet) or wok set over a high heat. Swirl the hot oil around the pan, then add the broccoli. Cover the pan and cook the broccoli for 3 minutes.

Meanwhile, toss together the onion, almonds and spices in a bowl. Stir the broccoli and reduce the heat to medium. A few lightly browned pieces are fine, but your aim is to keep the bright green colour, ensuring the broccoli is just tender. Add the onion mixture to the pan and stir through the broccoli. Cook for 5 minutes longer, stirring often.

Drizzle over the lime juice. Stir once as it sizzles, then immediately remove the pan from the heat and transfer its contents to a warm serving dish. Serve hot.

✳ **BROCCOLI** comes in many guises. In these recipes, use the type that is available to you, depending on where you are and the time of year. Each variety has its own texture, colour and flavour. After sampling many types, you will find your favourites. Try calabrese, purple sprouting, Tenderstem, romanesco and Italian leaf broccoli (sometimes called rapa, or broccoli rabe). Cauliflower is a good substitute if there is no type of broccoli is available.

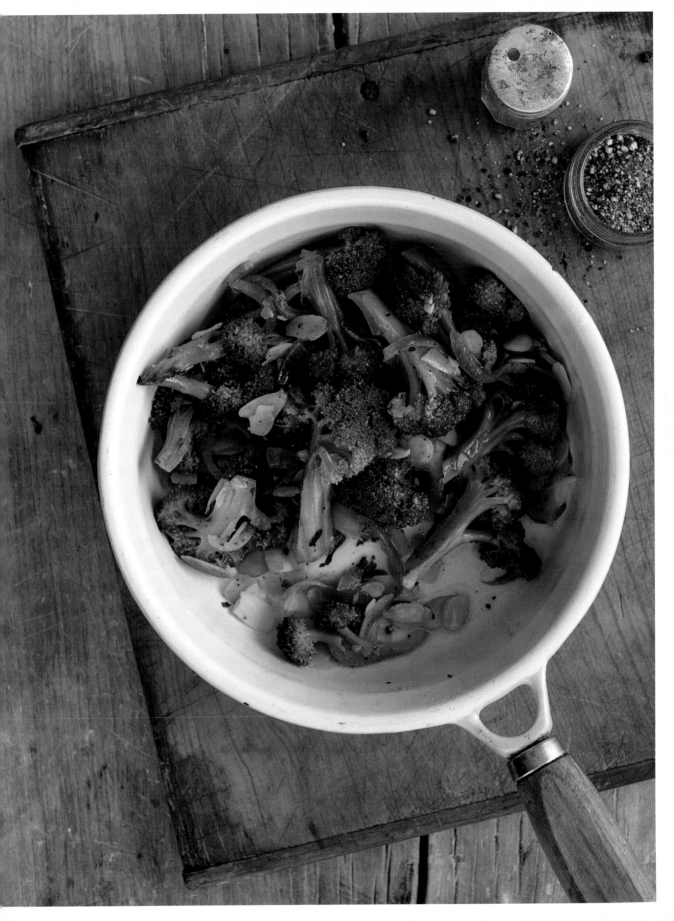

GREAT GRATED SALAD

You can make this slaw-like salad quickly, all by yourself – but it's more fun to play word games and think of tongue-twisters while you share the grater with your young ones. They will learn quickly and get better at it with practice. As we used to say, 'That grater was later a much greater grater!' Use this juicy combination of shredded veg to fill a baked potato, as a 'nest' for Sprouted Mung Beans (page 78), or serve alongside Mediterranean Spiced Rice and Lentils (page 130).

SERVES 4
PREPARATION TIME 15 MINUTES

1 medium carrot, grated

1 small turnip, grated

1 broccoli stalk (use the florets for another dish), peeled and grated

6 Brussels sprouts, grated

15g (½oz/about ½ cup) finely chopped fresh herbs such as basil, coriander (cilantro), lemon balm or flat-leaf parsley

Juice of 1 lemon

2 tablespoons extra virgin olive oil

1 tablespoon grated fresh ginger

1 red onion, quartered and thinly sliced

¼ teaspoon black pepper

¼ teaspoon salt, or to taste

OPTIONS AND VARIATIONS

You could grate the heart of a cabbage instead of the broccoli stalk, or peel and grate a small kohlrabi instead of the turnip. For a sweet note, drizzle 1 teaspoon barley malt or maple syrup over your portion.

Mix together all the ingredients in a bowl. Leave the salad to stand for a few minutes, then stir again. The vegetables will release some juices; aim to distribute these by stirring well before serving.

✱ GRATE SECRETS I used to throw away broccoli stalks and cabbage cores, until I discovered they are rather tasty – and highly nutritious, too. Peel away the thick, rough skin of the broccoli stalk to reveal the pale, tender heart, before grating (it is wonderful to bite into, too!). A cabbage core is similarly unpromising, but it does not need peeling and is crisper than the broccoli. Grate (or thinly slice it for other dishes) before use.

PRECIOUS GREENS

It is easy to bring seasonal greens together in one dish. As well as enjoying them at their best, bursting with fresh flavours, you'll benefit from the generous levels of nutrients in-season greens provide. Often, they supply just the nutrients you most need at that time of year. Serve your seasonal greens hot over grains, alongside a potato dish, and with a sauce or dressing of your choice.

SERVES 4

PREPARATION TIME 30 MINUTES

1 tablespoon untoasted sesame oil

At least 3 different types of seasonal greens and additional herbs selected from the lists below

Pour the oil into a large saucepan. Pick at least three different types of greens in addition to the herbs you want to use, and chop or slice the greens to create variety in their texture. Herbs should be trimmed of their coarse or woody stalks, then finely chopped. Press the greens and herbs into the pan in the order given (first on the list, first in the pan). Aim to absolutely fill the pan.

Cover the pan and cook over a medium heat for 12–15 minutes until the greens are tender but bright, stirring once or twice in that time.

SEASONAL GREENS

SPRING	SUMMER	AUTUMN	WINTER
Spring cabbage	Cabbage	Curly kale	Savoy cabbage
Cavolo nero	Chard (silver beet) or spinach	Cabbage	Turnip greens
Chicory	Broccoli	Brussels sprouts	Cauliflower
Tatsoi or pak choi (bok choy)	Pak choi (bok choy) or tatsoi	Beetroot (beet) greens	Kalettes (kale sprouts)
Purple sprouting broccoli	Asparagus	Leeks	Romanesco
Herbs: parsley, basil, oregano	Herbs: fennel, chives, chervil	Herbs: thyme, sage, marjoram	Herbs: parsley, rosemary, dried herbs

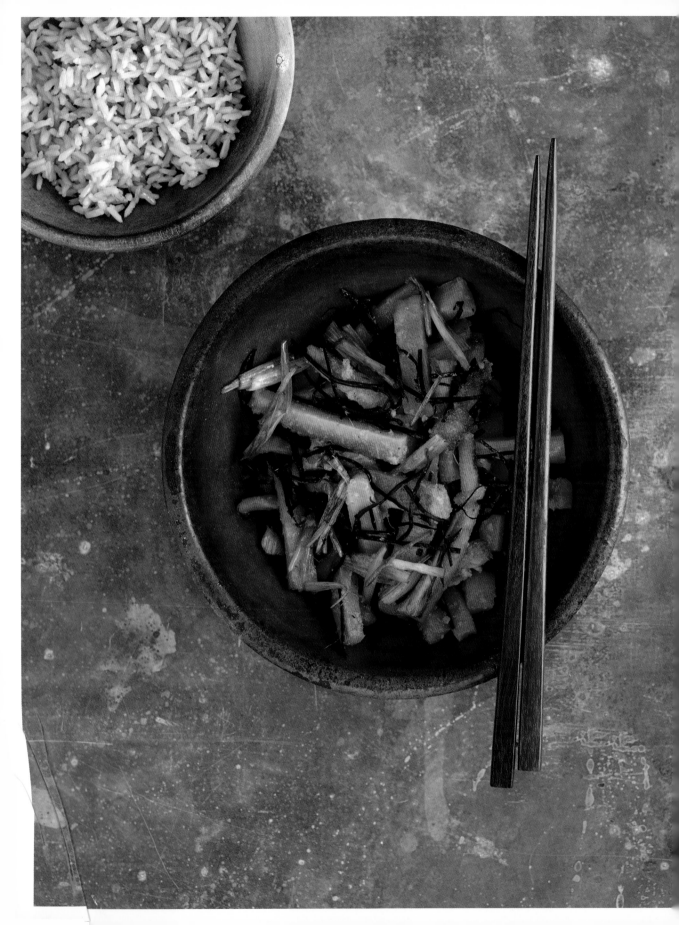

CARROT, ARAME AND GINGER SAUTÉ

Arame brings its unique flavour and delicate texture to the classic blend of carrot and ginger. I like to serve this with a selection of other equally colourful dishes, all of which work well together on the plate, allowing each person to serve themselves. For a simpler meal, serve with Broccoli Almond Sizzle (page190) and a portion of Three-grain Risotto (page 184).

SERVES 4

PREPARATION TIME 30 MINUTES

5g (⅛oz) dried arame

1 tablespoon untoasted sesame oil

4 medium carrots, sliced into sticks

4 spring onions (scallions), quartered along their length then cut into 8cm (3¼in) strips

2 tablespoons grated fresh ginger

¼ teaspoon black pepper

OPTIONS AND VARIATIONS

Add chopped garlic, to taste, when you add the spring onion.

Measure the arame into a bowl, cover with cold water and soak for 10 minutes.

Pour the oil into a large frying pan (skillet) set over a medium heat and add the carrot sticks. Cover the pan and cook for 5 minutes.

Add the spring onions, ginger and pepper, and stir well. Cover the pan and cook for 2–3 minutes.

Lift the arame out of its soaking water into a sieve and rinse under cold water. Drain and lay the arame on top of the other ingredients in the pan. Cover the pan and cook for about 5 minutes.

Remove the cover and cook for a final 2–3 minutes, stirring gently. Serve hot.

BEANSPROUT AND NOODLE CHAOS

There are no straight lines in this dish – everything gets in a tangle, hence the name. Crinkly dried eggless noodles, often sold in blocks, add to the tangle. This dish is easy to eat with chopsticks or a fork, and is ideal when you need a hot meal almost immediately. Serve with a side of Tempeh Crisps in Pomegranate Glaze (page 167) and some tamari or Japanese ume shiso seasoning to sprinkle over.

SERVES 4

PREPARATION TIME 20 MINUTES

15g (½oz) dried arame

1 tablespoon untoasted sesame oil

200g (7oz) thinly sliced greens, such as spring (collard) greens, cavolo nero, tatsoi, pak choi (bok choy) or chard (silver beet)

1 large carrot, grated

2 tablespoons grated orange zest

3 tablespoons grated fresh ginger

1 red chilli, thinly sliced

125g (4½oz) eggless dried noodles, preferably those sold in 'crinkled' blocks, broken into 8–10cm (3¼–4in) pieces

1 medium red onion, quartered and thinly sliced

250ml (9fl oz/1 cup) mung bean sprouts (see Sprouted Mung Beans, page 78)

OPTIONS AND VARIATIONS

Add chopped garlic, to taste. Use freshly squeezed orange juice instead of the water (if needed), toward the end of cooking. The carrot can be 'spiralized' instead of grated, if you have the gadget.

Put the arame in a bowl and cover with cold water. Leave to soak while you prepare the other ingredients.

It is best to have all the vegetables prepared before you start to cook. Pour the oil into a wok or large pan set over a medium-high heat. Add the greens, carrot, orange zest, ginger and chilli. Cover the pan and cook for 5 minutes.

Lift the arame out of its soaking water into a sieve. Rinse under cold water, then drain and add to the pan. Add the broken noodles and stir. Cover the pan and cook for 5 minutes. Add the onion and bean sprouts. Stir well and cover the pan once more.

After 2 minutes, check to see whether the noodles are cooked – you want them to be just tender. If necessary, add 1–2 tablespoons water, immediately cover the pan and cook a further minute or so. Take care not to overcook the noodles and sprouts – this dish should not be oily or soggy.

Serve the Chaos in wide, shallow bowls.

✳ **ARAME SEAWEED** has a delicate, lacy texture, with a mild but distinctive flavour unique to sea vegetables. Arame will cook quickly if it has been soaked in cold water for about 5 minutes. I've found it's best to lift the soaked arame out of its water first, rather than draining it directly through a sieve. This way, any grit is left behind in the bottom of the bowl (instead of being caught by the sieve).

FENNEL AND CITRUS TANGO

I never know quite how to categorize this flavoursome dish: is it a sauce or a salad? It can accompany salads and hot meals alike, by the bowlful or spoonful. I can use it immediately, store it in the refrigerator for tomorrow, or give the flavours a chance to develop and the vegetables time to soften slightly. Once, a family member was spotted having it for breakfast with some very crispy toast. Try it with Broccoli Almond Sizzle (page 90) and Three-Grain Risotto (page 184).

SERVES 4

PREPARATION TIME 15 MINUTES

4 layers of fennel (finocchio) bulb, very, very thinly sliced

1 medium carrot, grated

1 small red onion, quartered and thinly sliced

1 tablespoon chopped lemon balm

1 tablespoon chopped mint

2 segments from a peeled lemon (see note)

2 segments from a peeled orange (see note)

OPTIONS AND VARIATIONS

Add a pinch of cayenne pepper, sprinkled over the dish before serving. This dish is 'self-dressed' with citrus juices, but if you want to vary the flavours and build up more of a dressing, add a sprinkling of rice wine vinegar and a teaspoon of olive oil.

Toss the fennel, carrot, onion and herbs together in a serving bowl.

Slice the lemon and orange segments across their width, to make triangular shapes. Turn these, and any juice from them, into the serving bowl. Stir well, pressing the ingredients a little with the spoon as you mix.

Serve, or chill and serve.

✳ **PEELING CITRUS** An easy way to peel a lemon is to slice off its top and tail to reveal the pattern of segments. Then slice through the peel from the top to the tail by starting in line with one of the segment edges you see. Do that again but two segments along, then push your thumb under the peel and pull that two-segment wide piece of peel away. Now push your thumb into the end of the lemon and pull those segments away. You can use the same method for oranges, too.

CHICKPEA AND RUBY CHARD HUBBUB

I use a pressure cooker to cook the chickpeas (garbanzo beans) because they must be very tender. When I can find them, I use the especially large chickpeas, labelled 'extra' – they swell up almost to the size of a marble! A bed of couscous or plain basmati rice offers an appealing contrast to the warm colours of this dish. Serve your portion with a dollop of Margarita Yogurt Dip (page 90) and a spoonful of Sweetcorn and Pepper Relish (page 134) on the side.

SERVES 4

PREPARATION TIME 1 HOUR +

TIME TO SOAK THE CHICKPEAS

300g (10½oz/½ cup) dried chickpeas (garbanzo beans), washed and soaked for 8–12 hours (see How to Cook Beans, page 64)

10cm (4in) strip of kombu, rinsed

1 tablespoon untoasted sesame oil

1 whole garlic bulb, cloves separated and chopped

1 medium onion, finely chopped

½ teaspoon black pepper

½ teaspoon ground cinnamon

¼ teaspoon ground nutmeg

¼ teaspoon ground cloves

300g (10½oz) ruby chard (silver beet), sliced

1 small beetroot (beet), grated

OPTIONS AND VARIATIONS

This dish is not hot with spices – but if you would prefer something spicier, try doubling the black pepper or replacing it with fresh chilli or chilli flakes, to taste.

Drain and rinse the soaked chickpeas. Put the strip of kombu in the bottom of the pressure cooker, and tip the rinsed chickpeas on top. Add enough water to reach half the depth of the pan. Cover, seal and pressure-cook for 30 minutes.

Meanwhile, pour the oil into a large saucepan and sauté the garlic, onion and spices over a low heat for 5 minutes, stirring often. Add the chard and grated beetroot, and continue cooking, covered, over a low heat for 7–10 minutes until the vegetables are softened. Remove the pan from the heat and set aside until the chickpeas are cooked.

When the chickpeas are cooked, drain them and discard the kombu (if it hasn't dissolved), then turn the chickpeas into the pan with the chard mixture. Stir well. Return to a medium heat if you wish, until the dish is heated through.

Serve hot or cold.

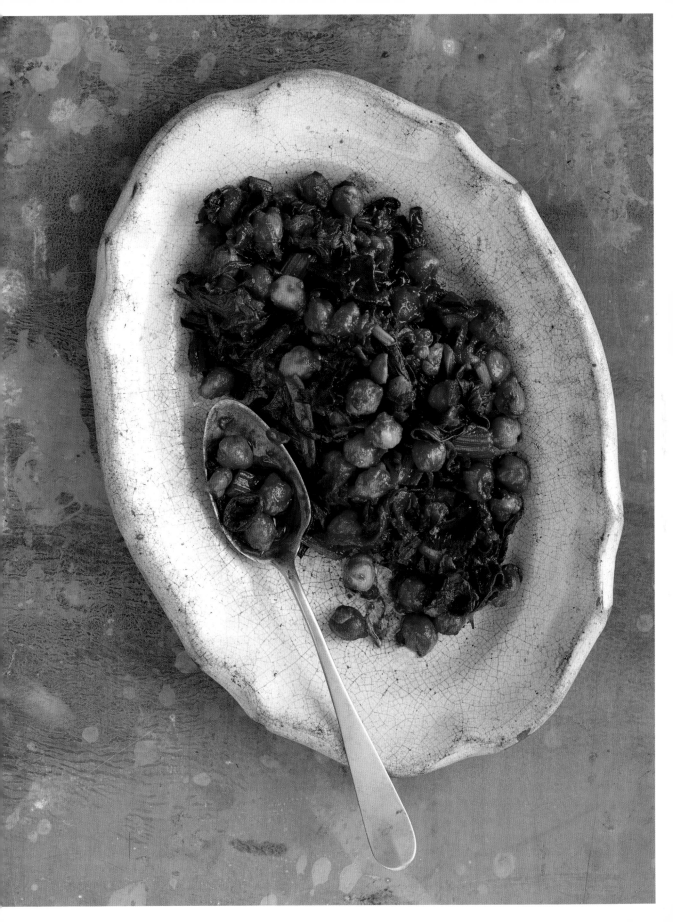

LENTILS IN WINTER SOUP

Frost will sweeten the flavour of most roots. Here, the parsnip and carrots deliver their wintry sweetness to the earthy flavour of lentils. For this soup, I prefer a chunky texture rather than a smooth purée, but whichever you choose won't affect the delicious flavour. I like to serve this with slices of Splendid Wholesome Loaf (page 120) and a small pot of Ginger and Nori Dressing (page 119), to dip the crust into. This simple, homely combination makes a robust meal.

SERVES 4

PREPARATION TIME 1 HOUR

1 tablespoon untoasted sesame oil

2 medium carrots, cut into coins

1 medium parsnip, cut into coins

2 medium onions, finely chopped

1 whole garlic bulb, cloves separated and chopped

10cm (4in) strip of kombu, rinsed

½ teaspoon Chinese five-spice

½ teaspoon black pepper

250g (9oz/1¼ cups) split red lentils

¼ teaspoon ground turmeric

OPTIONS AND VARIATIONS

Add 1 teaspoon vegan bouillon powder at the start of cooking, or ½ teaspoon dried basil when adding the ground turmeric.

Pour the oil into a large stockpot or saucepan set over a medium heat. Add the carrots, parsnip, onions, garlic, kombu, five-spice powder and black pepper. Cover the pan and leave to cook for 15 minutes, stirring once in that time.

Meanwhile, measure the lentils into a bowl and cover with water. Stir them around a little, then drain away the water. Repeat this procedure twice more until the water runs clear.

When the vegetables have had their 15 minutes, add the lentils, stir well and pour in enough water to fully cover the contents of the pan. Cover and leave to cook for 15 minutes. Stir now and then, adding more water if needed as the lentils swell and absorb liquid.

When the lentils and vegetables are fully tender, remove the kombu (if you wish), then use a hand-held blender to purée the mixture to the texture you prefer. Add a little more water if needed.

Stir in the ground turmeric, then stir well and bring to a low simmer. Cover the pan and remove from the heat a few minutes before serving. Leave the soup to stand for 2 hours to deepen the flavour, or put it in the refrigerator if you wish to serve it later today or tomorrow.

✳ **KOMBU SEAWEED** adds minerals to the nutrient value of soups and stews. But I 'found' it because I am always interested to learn of methods or ingredients that can bring flavours together, in soups especially. Kombu has a subtle umami flavour, similar to bouillon, and a definite unifying effect. I rinse it first, then simply drop it into the pot. The kombu sometimes dissolves during cooking – if it doesn't, I just remove it before serving.

SIMPLE RED LENTIL DHAL

Red lentils are inexpensive, quick to cook, very nutritious and easy to digest. You can turn them into soups, pâté or something like this dish, which humbly acknowledges the cuisines of other lands. Be creative; experiment with different combinations and quantities of spices. Make this early in the day, or the day before you want to serve it. Store it in the refrigerator, then reheat and serve with plain rice and a side dish of Dressed Greens and Beans (page 154) and All-Day Chutney (page 247).

SERVES 4

PREPARATION TIME 1 HOUR

250g (9oz/1¼ cups) split red lentils

1 tablespoon coconut oil

1 whole garlic bulb, cloves separated and chopped

1 fresh chilli, finely chopped

1 teaspoon vegan bouillon powder

1 teaspoon cumin seeds

½ teaspoon ground cinnamon

½ teaspoon ground ginger

½ teaspoon ground allspice

½ teaspoon ground coriander

½ teaspoon ground turmeric

3 tablespoons chopped fresh coriander (cilantro) leaves

OPTIONS AND VARIATIONS

Use ½ teaspoon chilli flakes instead of the fresh chilli. Add 1 tablespoon dried basil instead of the fresh coriander (cilantro) leaves.

Pour the lentils into a large saucepan and cover with cold water. Stir well, and drain the murky water away through a sieve. Leave the lentils in the sieve and rinse them under cold running water.

Tip the lentils back into the rinsed pan, and cover with fresh water to about twice their depth. Set the pan over a medium-high heat and bring the contents to a near-simmer. Reduce the heat to low, cover the pan and simmer gently for about 20 minutes.

Meanwhile, in a separate pan set over a low heat, melt the coconut oil and add the garlic, chilli, bouillon powder, cumin seeds, cinnamon, ginger, allspice and ground coriander. Cover and leave to cook, stirring once or twice, for 10 minutes.

Stir the lentils every now and then, and add more water if needed – the aim is to cook them down to a purée. Once the lentils are soft and have lost their shape, leave them over a low heat while you finish the spice mixture.

Add the turmeric and fresh coriander to the pan of spices. Stir over the heat for 1–2 minutes, then tip the spice mixture into the cooked lentils. Immediately ladle some cooked lentils into the empty spice pan, stirring to collect any spicy flavours, then tip these lentils back into the main pan.

Stir the dhal over the low heat to distribute the spices. Both the turmeric and the lentils themselves will cause the dhal to thicken.

Cover the pan, remove from the heat and set aside so that the flavours can blend. Reheat as necessary to serve hot, adding more water if necessary to give the consistency you desire.

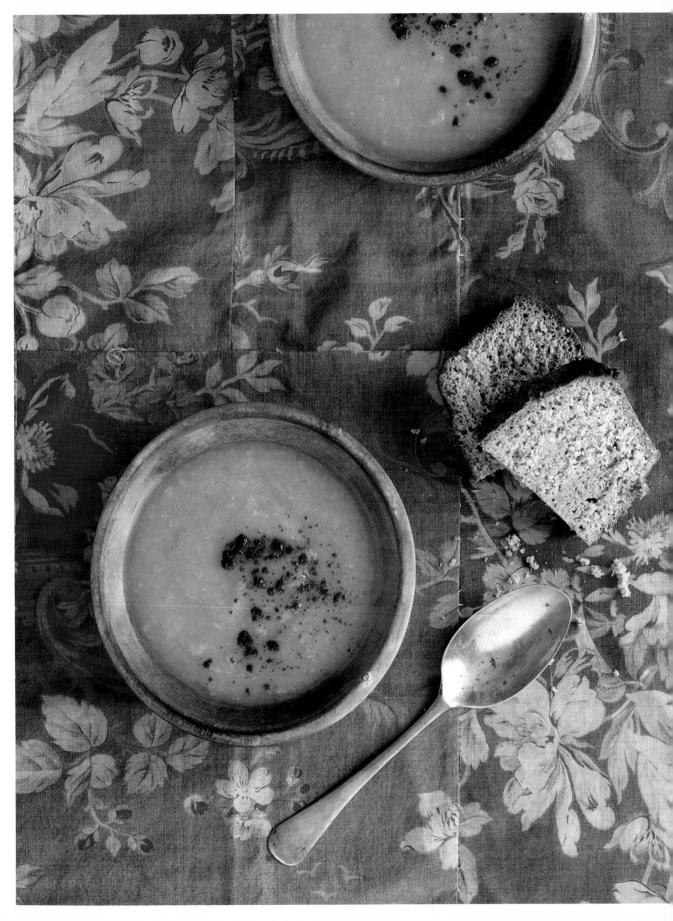

PUMPKIN AND PARSNIP SOUP

Pumpkin can be a strong, earthy flavour. In this soup, the parsnip moves the flavour to a sweeter note. I make this soup in the autumn (fall), after the first frosts have enriched the sugars in the parsnips. I often double the recipe and freeze some for use later in the year. A steamed pumpkin of any size can easily make two meals – so sometimes I make this soup by using up some pumpkin left over from a previous meal. A slice of Seeded Spelt Bread (page 87) spread with Herb and Onion Bean Butter (page 71) is a great accompaniment.

SERVES 4

PREPARATION TIME 1 HOUR

½ small to medium pumpkin, quartered and deseeded, but left unpeeled

1 tablespoon untoasted sesame oil

2 large onions, chopped

1 large parsnip, finely chopped

½ teaspoon Chinese five-spice

¼ teaspoon black pepper

1 litre (35fl oz/4 cups) vegetable stock or water

OPTIONS AND VARIATIONS

If you use water instead of vegetable stock, you can add 1 teaspoon vegan bouillon powder with the spices.

Put the raw pumpkin quarters, skin side up, in a steamer basket set over simmering water. Cover the pan and steam for 10–15 minutes.

Lift the hot quarters onto a chopping board to cool a little. They might break apart, but don't worry.

Meanwhile, pour the oil into a large saucepan set over a medium heat Add the onions and parsnip, cover the pan and sauté for 15 minutes, stirring occasionally. When the onions and parsnip are tender, add the five-spice powder and black pepper. Stir and cook a further 2 minutes.

Scoop the steamed pumpkin flesh from the pumpkin skin, and add to the mixture in the pan. Add the stock and stir well. Purée the mixture using a hand-held blender, leaving a few chunks of parsnip and onion. The soup will thicken. Add more stock or water if you wish, to create your preferred consistency.

Cover the pan and bring the soup to a low simmer. Remove from the heat and serve immediately; or set aside to cool, then refrigerate to allow the flavours to mature, and serve the next day.

HOMECOMING STEW

You rarely hear anyone talk about stews, yet they are fantastically versatile and nutritious. Warming and enticingly aromatic, they can sustain even the hungriest young person. They create a homey feeling, and I love to offer a bowlful to visitors – they always say, 'Yes!' Serve in a bowl all by itself, or ladle onto hot couscous, with a side dish of Dressed Greens and Beans (page 154).

MAKES 8 BOWLFULS

PREPARATION TIME 1¼ HOURS

4 tablespoons untoasted sesame oil

2 medium onions, chopped

2 medium carrots, chopped

2 medium potatoes, chopped

2 medium turnips, chopped

2 celery stalks, finely chopped

1 small swede (rutabaga), chopped

100g (3½oz/½ cup) split red lentils, rinsed and drained

2 tablespoons plain (all-purpose) flour

2 teaspoons dried basil

1 teaspoon dried oregano

½ teaspoon black pepper

½ teaspoon ground turmeric

750ml (26fl oz/3 cups) vegetable stock or water or oat milk

6 large sprigs of fresh flat-leaf parsley, finely chopped

2 outer leaves of cabbage, finely chopped

OPTIONS AND VARIATIONS

You could add 750ml (26fl oz/ 3 cups) tomato passata (purée) instead of the stock – if you choose this option, omit the flour and ground turmeric, but include the herbs and black pepper.

Pour half of the oil into a large saucepan, and arrange the onions in the bottom of the pan. Add layers of carrot, potato, turnip, celery, swede and lentils, in that order. Cover the pan and set it over a high heat for 5 minutes. Reduce the heat to medium and cook, undisturbed, for a further 15 minutes.

Meanwhile, mix together the flour, dried herbs, black pepper and turmeric in a small bowl. Pour the remaining oil into another saucepan set over a low to medium heat. Add the flour mixture; stir so that the oil is absorbed and the flour mixture is cooked, to create a firm paste. Add the stock to this saucepan, a little at a time, constantly stirring over a low to medium heat. The stock will be absorbed into the flour mixture, which in turn will thicken the stock.

Add the parsley and cabbage to the stew saucepan, and carefully stir. Pour the thickened stock over the ingredients in the stew pan, stir well and cover the pan. Adjust the heat if needed, and stir from time to time as it cooks over a low to medium heat for a further 45 minutes. When all the ingredients are tender, remove from the heat.

Serve hot.

WHITE BEAN SOUP

Creamy and pastel-coloured, this soup looks delicate but is very sustaining. Use any white beans, such as cannellini or butter (lima) beans, and include the green part of the leeks to give a lovely green tint. I've also made this with chickpeas (garbanzo beans), which benefit from simmering in the soup for a little longer than other beans. Excellent with a Kohlrabi and Cucumber Sandwich (page 123) or a toasted slice of Four-Day Sourdough Bread (page 118).

SERVES 4

PREPARATION TIME 45 MINUTES

1 tablespoon untoasted sesame oil

1 small white potato, cubed

2 medium onions, finely chopped

2 leeks, chopped

1 teaspoon vegan bouillon powder

1 teaspoon dried basil

½ teaspoon dried oregano

½ teaspoon black pepper

250g (9oz) cooked white beans such as cannellini or butter (lima) beans (see How to Cook Beans, page 64)

OPTIONS AND VARIATIONS

If your leeks don't have a green portion, add 4 tablespoons chopped flat-leaf parsley to the pan before you purée the soup. Add ¼ teaspoon crushed caraway seeds when you begin to cook the potato.

Put the oil in a large saucepan set over a medium heat. Add the potato, onions and leeks, cover the pan and cook for 20 minutes, stirring occasionally.

When the vegetables are tender, add the bouillon powder, herbs and black pepper, and stir well. Add 1 litre (35fl oz/4 cups) water, and use a hand-held blender to purée the soup.

Add the white beans, reduce the heat and cover the pan. Bring to a low simmer, and remove from the heat before serving.

✳ **A BRIGHTER SHADE OF GREEN** There is just a hint of green in this soup, but at certain times of year the soup can look too pale. A quick fix is to add the merest amount of ground turmeric (⅛ teaspoon) and stir it into the hot broth. It will bring out, or 'brighten', the green in the ingredients and boost the visual appeal. Use this tip for other recipes to boost the brightness.

SEAWEED AND POTATO CUTLETS

I first made these with steamed potatoes, left over from the previous day, that had spent the night in the refrigerator. The arame suddenly seemed like a perfect match, so I got to work. These are filling and satisfying, and can be made into any shape you like: I've tried wedges, quarter-rounds and rectangles, and they all work. Family members tend to make big round patties, which are easy to handle. The turmeric gives a little colour and added body. Have a cutlet with Great Grated Salad (page 192) and Tempeh Crisps in Pomegranate Glaze (page 167).

SERVES 4

PREPARATION TIME 40 MINUTES

10g (¼oz) dried arame

4 medium potatoes, cooked

60ml (2fl oz/¼ cup) plant milk or vegetable stock

60ml (2fl oz/¼ cup) untoasted sesame oil

4 garlic cloves, finely chopped

1 teaspoon black pepper

½ teaspoon caraway seeds, lightly crushed

4 tablespoons plain (all-purpose) or wholemeal (whole-wheat) flour

1 tablespoon dried oregano

½ teaspoon ground turmeric

OPTIONS AND VARIATIONS

For a stronger sea-vegetable flavour, add 2 teaspoons nori flakes to the flour mixture.

Soak the arame in a bowl of cold water, and set aside.

Remove any skins from the cooked potatoes, and roughly chop them into a large bowl. Add the plant milk, and use a fork to create a rough-textured mash.

Heat 1 tablespoon of the oil in a frying pan (skillet) over a medium heat. Add the garlic, ½ teaspoon of the black pepper and the caraway seeds. When they start to sizzle, lift the soaked arame from the soaking water onto the chopping board. Chop the strands in half and add to the garlic and spices in the pan. Cover the pan, reduce the heat and cook for 5 minutes. Remove from the heat, and tip the cooked garlic and arame mixture into the potato mash mixture. Stir well.

Mix together the flour, oregano, turmeric and remaining black pepper in a small bowl. Sprinkle a little of the flour mixture onto a chopping board. Put a quarter of the potato mixture onto the floured board. Dampen your hands or two wooden spoons, and shape the mixture into a cutlet. Press the cutlet edges to neaten them, and sprinkle the top with more of the seasoned flour.

Let the cutlets stand for a few minutes before cooking – this will help them to hold their shape when they are fried.

Using the same frying pan, add a little of the remaining oil and set the pan over a medium heat. Add the first cutlet. Cover the pan and cook the cutlet on one side for about 5 minutes until golden and lightly crusted. Turn the cutlet over and cook the other side, leaving the pan uncovered.

Put the cooked cutlet on a plate, and keep warm in a low oven while you repeat this process for the other cutlets.

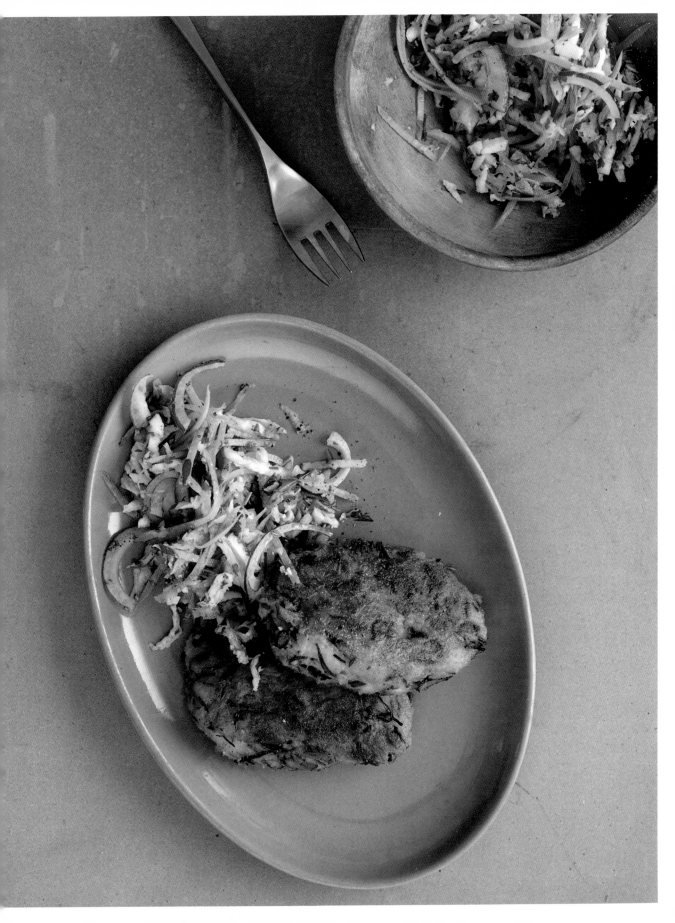

GRAVY OF THE GODS

Almost everyone loves gravy served over a mound of roast vegetables, such as in Roast Dinner Medley (page 175), or served with Shepherd's Garden Pie (page 210). Read the labels of brand-name gravy powders: some of these contain animal-based ingredients, while, sadly, some plant-based products are processed in factories that also process animal-based products.

MAKES 500ML (2 CUPS)

PREPARATION TIME 30 MINUTES

2 tablespoons untoasted sesame oil

1 medium onion, finely chopped

4 garlic cloves, finely chopped

½ teaspoon dried oregano

¼ teaspoon black pepper

Pinch of dried thyme or crushed rosemary

3 tablespoons vegan gravy powder

OPTIONS AND VARIATIONS

If you don't have gravy powder, use 3 tablespoons plain cornflour (cornstarch) instead – but note that this gravy will not be as brown. For a brown gravy using cornflour, cook the onions at a higher temperature to brown them, but without letting them become crisp; or stir in 1 tablespoon vegetable stock concentrate or yeast extract just before serving.

Pour the oil into a small saucepan and set over a low to medium heat. Add the onion, cover the pan and cook until very tender, about 15 minutes. Aim to soften the onion, almost to the point of caramelization. Next, add the garlic, oregano and black pepper, and cook for 5 minutes, stirring often.

Meanwhile, put the gravy powder in a measuring jug (large measuring cup), and add 2 tablespoons water. Stir to make a paste, then gradually add enough water to make the volume up to 500ml (17fl oz/2 cups), stirring well.

When the garlic is softened, gradually add the liquid mixture to the saucepan. Keep stirring – the liquid will thicken and become gravy.

Serve hot.

✱ **MEDIAEVAL RE-ENACTMENT** is not for everyone but, like the fascination with dinosaurs or big trucks, it can have a powerful appeal to young people. A surprise visit by a familiar-looking group of very hungry young mediaeval travellers carrying cudgels and blunt swords resulted in this serving idea for the gravy. The 'trenchers' they requested were made from thick slices of wholemeal bread. Each was topped with a spoonful of cooked beans and a ladle of this gravy, steaming hot and aromatic. I was not sure they would approve, but they loved it and praised me for my research!

BABY CORN AND CARROTS WITH HERB AND GARLIC DRIZZLE

Prepare the dressing first, so that the flavours can blend. The corn and carrots are tiny and won't take long to cook. The sweetness from the date molasses in this dressing accentuates the natural sweetness of the young vegetables, rather than overwhelming them. Preparing the garlic in this way develops its mellow, buttery flavour – quite unlike the sharpness of raw garlic. Try the dressing with steamed asparagus or drizzled over Sprouted Mung Beans (page 78) or Entirely Green Salad (page 92).

SERVES 4

PREPARATION TIME 30 MINUTES

4 garlic cloves, coarsely chopped

½ teaspoon dried basil

¼ teaspoon dried oregano

Pinch of salt

Pinch of cayenne pepper

2 tablespoons apple cider vinegar

Juice of ½ lemon

60ml (2fl oz/¼ cup) extra virgin olive oil

½ teaspoon date molasses

250g (9oz) baby carrots

250g (9oz) baby sweetcorn

Put the garlic in a small saucepan with 4 tablespoons water. Cover and set the pan over a medium heat. Simmer for about 5 minutes until the garlic is tender enough to mash with a fork. Remove from the heat.

Stir together the herbs, salt, cayenne pepper, vinegar and lemon juice in a bowl, and add the cooked garlic and its juices. Stir well and ensure that the garlic is mashed thoroughly.

Add the olive oil and date molasses, and whisk everything together. Depending on the size of your lemon, you might need to adjust the amount of oil to create a fairly thick dressing.

Put the dressing aside for 10–15 minutes while you prepare the vegetables, to allow the flavours to mature.

Place the carrots in a steaming basket, and put the baby sweetcorn on top of them. Put the basket in a pan with water to a depth of about 3cm (1¼in), cover the pan and place over a medium heat. Steam the vegetables for about 7 minutes until they are just tender. Arrange on a serving plate, and drizzle with the dressing.

OPTIONS AND VARIATIONS

Use ¼ teaspoon dried thyme as a replacement for both the dried basil and oregano. Add 250g (9oz) baby courgettes (zucchini) to the steaming basket.

SHEPHERD'S GARDEN PIE

I love the crispy texture on the top of this dish and how it softens as the serving spoon digs deeper into it. That first scoop releases an aroma that quickly fills the kitchen. Some steamed Brussels sprouts or boiled green peas are all that you need as an accompaniment, though hungry people might like to add a sausage made from Quick Patty Cake Mix (page 50).

SERVES 4

PREPARATION TIME 1 HOUR 20 MINUTES

125g (4½oz/scant ⅔ cup) brown lentils, rinsed

4 medium potatoes, peeled and chopped

2 celery stalks, chopped

2 cabbage leaves, finely chopped

2 medium parsnips, finely chopped

2 medium carrots, grated or finely chopped

1 medium tomato, finely chopped

1 tablespoon untoasted sesame oil, plus extra for drizzling

1 large onion, chopped

1 teaspoon black pepper

½ teaspoon ground cinnamon

½ teaspoon oregano

½ teaspoon thyme

3 tablespoons vegan gravy powder

500ml (17fl oz/2 cups) vegetable stock or water

A little plant milk, for the mash

OPTIONS AND VARIATIONS

Greens such as celery leaf or kale can be chopped and added instead of cabbage.

Preheat the oven to 200°C (400°F).

Put the lentils in a heatproof bowl, cover with boiling water and set aside.

Steam the potatoes until tender, about 15 minutes.

In a wide 2-litre (70fl oz/8-cup) ovenproof dish, mix the celery, cabbage, parsnips, carrots and tomato until evenly distributed. Drain the lentils, rinse them, and drain again. Spoon them over the vegetables in the ovenproof dish.

Meanwhile, pour the 1 tablespoon sesame oil into a saucepan, and add the onion, black pepper, cinnamon and herbs. Sauté over a medium heat for about 10 minutes.

Mix the gravy powder into 100ml (3½fl oz/scant ½ cup) of the stock to make a paste. Stir in the remaining stock, and gradually add this mixture to the sautéed onions, stirring as the mixture thickens. After about 5 minutes, pour the gravy over the lentils in the ovenproof dish.

Mash the steamed potatoes, adding a little plant milk if necessary to make a soft, spreadable mash. Spread the mash over the pie.

Drizzle with a little oil, and bake in the oven for 45–50 minutes until the top is turning golden. Let stand for 10 minutes before serving.

WINTER SOLSTICE PIE

This warming, filling pie is unusual for its combination of ingredients. It is creamy-coloured, except for the spinach, but you can include different types of potato to add interest: strongly coloured varieties include Highland Burgundy Red, Violetta, Salad Blue, Vitelotte and Shetland Black. They're all flavoursome and would add a contrast in colour and texture. Don't try to slice this pie neatly – you need to slice the crust and spoon it out ... and then it likes to sprawl across the plate! Try it served with a winter version of Precious Greens (page 193) or Cabbage and Pink Salad (page 244).

SERVES 4

PREPARATION TIME 1 HOUR

500g (1lb 2oz) potatoes, peeled and thinly sliced

500g (1lb 2oz) onions, thinly sliced

Pinch of ground nutmeg

500g (1lb 2oz) apples, sliced

100g (3½oz) baby spinach, rinsed and drained

70ml (2¼ fl oz/scant ⅓ cup) untoasted sesame oil, plus extra for greasing the dish

70ml (2¼ fl oz/scant ⅓ cup) plant milk

2 teaspoons prepared mustard

½ quantity Vegan Shortcrust Pastry (page 265)

Salt and pepper, to taste

OPTIONS AND VARIATIONS

Add a little crushed caraway seed to the potato layers, or a pinch of cayenne pepper to the apple layers.

Preheat the oven to 180°C (350°F), and lightly oil a 2-litre (70fl oz/8-cup) ovenproof dish.

Layer the ingredients in this order: potato, onion, seasoning to taste; then apple. Repeat this pattern until all these ingredients have been used, then cover with the spinach.

Whisk together the oil, plant milk and mustard, and pour over the spinach.

Roll out the prepared pastry so that it is slightly larger than the dish. Carefully lay it over the filling, and tuck it round the edges to create a mound. Roll the overhanging pastry inwards, or crimp, to create an attractive rim.

Bake in the oven for 45–50 minutes until golden. Serve hot.

APPLE BASKET CAKE

The arrangement of the sliced apples that give this cake its distinctive surface texture is an opportunity for creativity – especially if you are being helped by a young cook. A spiral or concentric circles give a basketweave effect, but snowflakes, windmills and latticework are also possible. A slice of this goes perfectly with a spoonful of Apple Butter (page 143) and a mug of Choc Hotlate (page 171).

Preheat oven to 180°C (350°F), and lightly oil a 23cm (9in) cake pan.

Peel, core and slice the apples, dropping the slices into a bowl. Add the lemon juice and stir gently so that the apple slices are coated with juice, which will prevent them turning brown. Leave them in the juice until needed.

Mix together the flour, ½ teaspoon of the cinnamon, cayenne and baking powder in a large bowl.

In a jug (large measuring cup), dissolve 100g (3½oz/½ cup) of the brown sugar in the plant milk. Add the oil, tahini and vinegar, and whisk together. Drain the lemon juice from the sliced apples and whisk into this mixture. Stir the wet ingredients into the dry ones, and spread the batter in the pan.

Arrange the apple slices on top of the batter. Mix the remaining 50g (2oz/¼ cup) sugar and the remaining ½ teaspoon cinnamon in a small bowl. Sprinkle this mixture over the apples.

Bake in the oven for 20–25 minutes until the cake is risen and golden around the sunken apples. Cool, slice and serve.

MAKES 1 CAKE

PREPARATION TIME 40 MINUTES

2–4 medium apples

Juice of 1 lemon

400g (14oz/2⅔ cups) plain (all-purpose) or wholemeal (whole-wheat) flour

1 teaspoon ground cinnamon

¼ teaspoon cayenne pepper

2 tablespoons baking powder

150g (5½oz/¾ cup, lightly packed) soft light brown sugar

350ml (12fl oz/1½ cups) plant milk

90ml (3fl oz) untoasted sesame oil

60ml (2fl oz/¼ cup) tahini

1 tablespoon apple cider vinegar

OPTIONS AND VARIATIONS

Sprinkle a handful of flaked almonds over the apples, just before you sprinkle the cinnamon sugar.

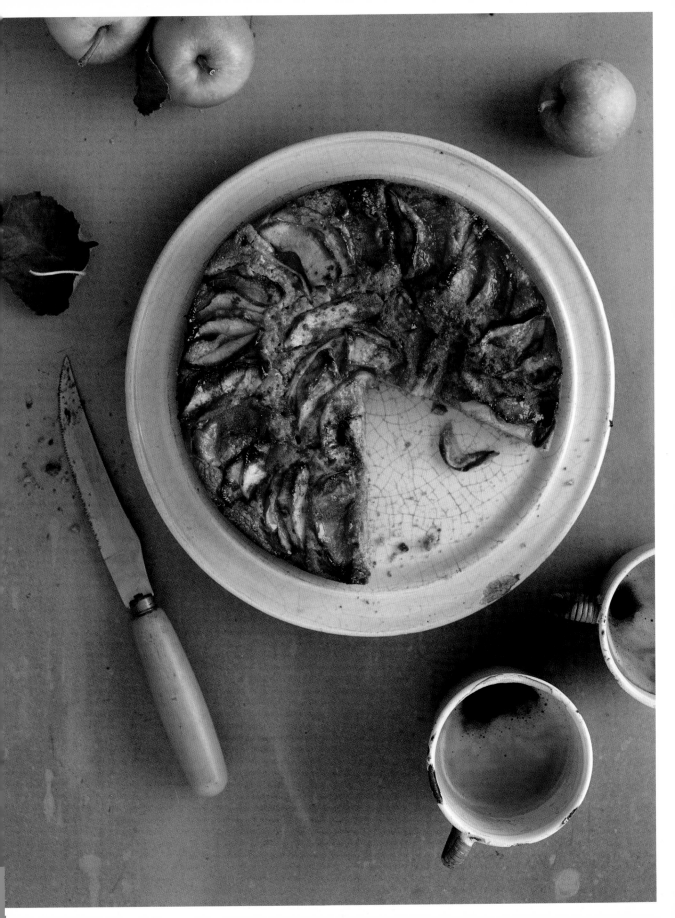

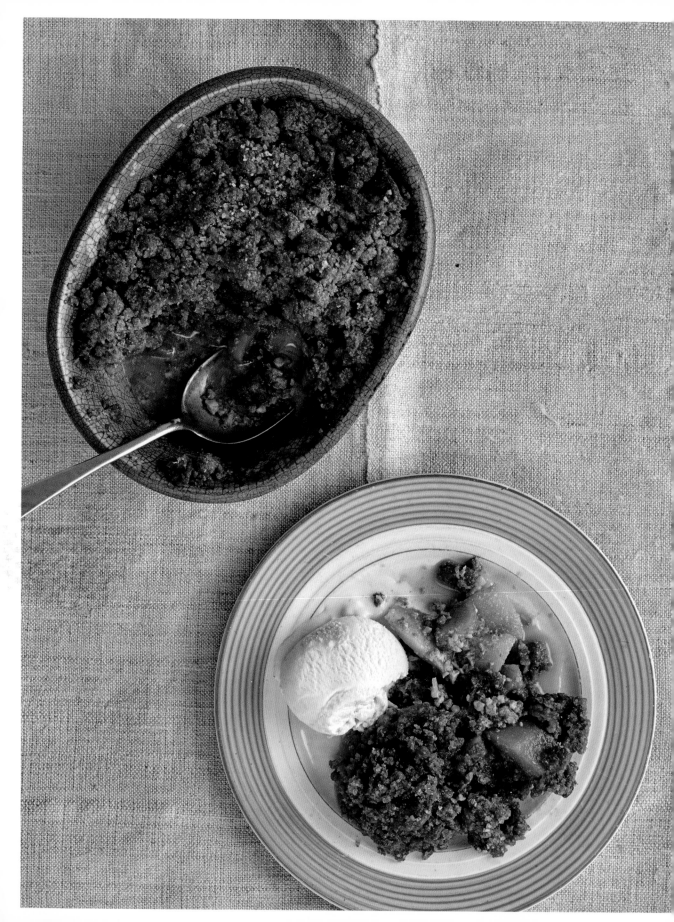

BAKED BARTLETT CRUMBLE

To my mind, Bartlett (Williams) pears are the iconic sun-kissed pear and represent lush abundance and hardiness in equal measure. They're often so big I don't know how the tree manages to hold them all. Usually, I simply bite into them, but this dish is a special treat. The idea is to fill the baking dish, so, if the pears you have are small, use three or four. A light drizzle of date molasses over each portion is delicious. A single wedge of Grilled Oranges with Maple Syrup (page 172), as a completely unnecessary accompaniment, accents the orange flavour baked into this dish.

SERVES 4

PREPARATION TIME 45 MINUTES

50g (1¾oz/½ cup) walnuts, crushed

2 Bartlett (Williams) pears

70ml (2¼fl oz) freshly squeezed orange juice

100g (3½oz/½ cup) soft light brown sugar

100g (3½oz/⅔ cup) plain (all-purpose) or wholemeal (whole-wheat) flour

½ teaspoon ground cinnamon

¼ teaspoon ground nutmeg

70g (2½oz) vegan margarine, plus extra for greasing the dish

OPTIONS AND VARIATIONS

I love this with the skin left on the pears, but it's your choice! Peel them if you wish.

Preheat the oven to 180°C (350°F), and lightly grease a 28cm (11¼in) pie dish with a little vegan margarine.

Sprinkle the crushed walnuts over the bottom of the pie dish. Core and slice the pears, and layer the slices on top of the walnuts. Pour over the orange juice.

In a bowl, mix together the sugar, flour and spices. Using a fork or your fingers, rub the margarine into the dry mixture to give a texture like fine breadcrumbs. Sprinkle the crumble mixture over the pears.

Bake in the oven for 30 minutes until the crumble topping is crisp.

BLUEBERRY APPLE PIE

Blueberries make a memorable pie. I use fresh berries – but I have to hide away just enough to make this so they aren't all eaten beforehand! Apple brings its sweetness and takes up the lovely juices from the berries as they cook. Its tender chunks create a texture contrast too. I like this served slightly warm, with a spoonful of soya ice cream.

MAKES 1 LARGE PIE

PREPARATION TIME 45 MINUTES

1 quantity Vegan Shortcrust Pastry (page 265)

2 medium apples

1kg (2¼lb) fresh blueberries

50g (1¾oz/¼ cup) granulated sugar

2 tablespoons plain (all-purpose) flour

OPTIONS AND VARIATIONS

Use 1 tablespoon oat bran instead of the flour.

Preheat the oven to 180°C (350°F). Line a 28cm (11¼in) pie dish with half of the pastry, and prepare the top crust.

Peel, core and slice the apples. Spread the apple slices over the bottom of the pastry base. Tip the blueberries into the pie dish, and spread evenly to cover the apples.

Mix together the sugar and flour in a small bowl, and sprinkle the mixture evenly over the berries.

Position the prepared top crust over the pie, seal together the edges of the pastry and pierce the top crust with a fork or knife.

Bake for 25–30 minutes until the pastry is golden and crisp.

Cool and serve.

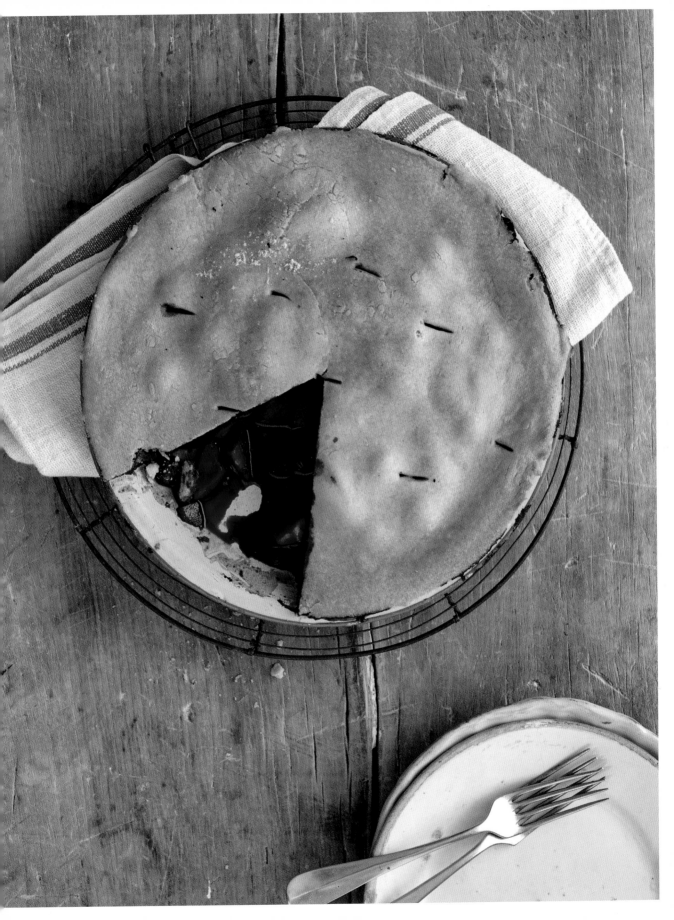

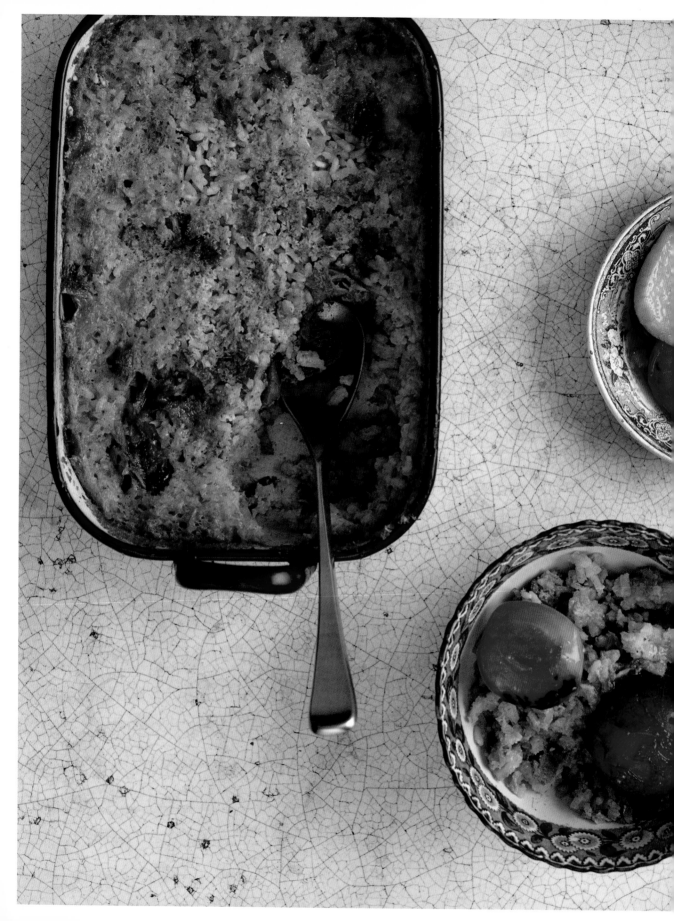

RICE PUDDING WITH COCONUT AND CHOPPED DATES

This luscious treat makes a comforting conclusion to a long, late dinner. Serve warm or cold – and consider cooking a double batch because it makes a lovely breakfast, too. As there is no added sugar – only the sweetness of the spices and fruit – some might want a little maple or barley malt syrup drizzled over their portion.

SERVES 4

PREPARATION TIME 1 HOUR

2 tablespoons coconut oil

50g (1¾oz/½ cup) desiccated (shredded) coconut

100g (3½oz/½ cup) dried dates, finely chopped

200g (7oz/scant 1 cup) pudding or arborio rice

500ml (17fl oz/2 cups) coconut or soya milk

¼ teaspoon ground cinnamon

¼ teaspoon ground ginger

¼ teaspoon ground nutmeg

OPTIONS AND VARIATIONS

This makes a luscious, tender pudding that stands in the dish. If you prefer a more creamy texture, add another 100ml (3½fl oz/scant ½ cup) milk at the start of cooking. Use finely chopped dried apricots instead of the dates.

Preheat the oven to 200°C (400°F).

Use half of the coconut oil to coat a 1-litre (35fl oz/4-cup) ovenproof dish (one with a lid). Sprinkle the desiccated coconut over the oiled surface, including the sides as much as possible. Aim for a layer of desiccated coconut about 1cm (½in) thick over the bottom of the dish.

Arrange the chopped dates over the coconut, then sprinkle the rice evenly over the dates. Dot the remaining coconut oil over the top of the rice.

Measure the milk into a jug (large measuring cup), and whisk the spices into it until they are evenly mixed. Pour the spiced milk over the rice and cover the dish.

Bake in the oven for 5 minutes, then reduce the oven temperature to 150°C (300°F) and cook for a further 55 minutes. For a crisp topping, uncover the dish and bake for 5 minutes more.

Let the pudding sit for a few minutes before serving, or allow it to cool completely.

✳ **AN OCCASIONAL TREAT** This recipe is one that remains in the 20 per cent part of my diet! I think it will always be there: it uses white arborio rice and, despite that, I am likely to have it once or twice each year. But don't let me tempt you …

THINKING DEEPER

RED IN TOOTH AND CLAW

You never hear anyone say: 'Nature, gloriously green,' or 'Nature, blue of lake and sky.' Instead, people repeat a line from Tennyson, 'Nature, red in tooth and claw,' and assume it must be true.

Following the death of a dear friend, Alfred Tennyson wrote *In Memoriam*, in which he lamented the cruelty of Nature. In his poem he is clearly grieving; he wants to rail at *someone*. And so his Nature, personified as female, is violent, cruel and uncaring. The fact that this imagery has endured for so long is proof that he was a good wordsmith. But was Tennyson correct in his assessment?

Nowadays, his words are often used to explain away actions that are performed *against* the natural world. Hunting, trapping, fishing and destruction of forests are clear examples — but so are bullying, social cruelty and patterns of behaviour that are intended to harm or dominate others. If a person mumbles Tennyson's phrase, they can feel justified: what they've done is okay because, well, it's natural. They had to do it to the other before the other did it to them. It's rather like having your cake and eating it, too: claiming to be part of the natural order and, in the same moment, directly opposing it.

This is not quite thinking. It is learning by rote without really learning at all. The phrase and the behaviour are repeated without question and passed on. Like an inoculation, it leaves its dose of toxicity. Fear of Nature is one toxin; a sense of separateness is another. Ultimately, the jab inspires a combative relationship with Nature. No wonder we are in a pickle.

Nature is infinitely ordered, although sometimes we cannot or will not see that fact. It would be soothing to say here that Nature is patient, but perhaps 'enduring' is more accurate. Nature is responsive and, while there certainly have been catastrophes for some species, Nature's responses are both creative and adaptive. How could it be otherwise? Nature is one entire, living complexity. It is old; 'she' is old and vast and powerful. There is a lot for her to look after!

At some point in the past, well before Tennyson, our species pitted itself against Nature, exercising coercive, bully-boy tactics to make the natural world do what we wanted. In an intoxication of ignorance and arrogance, not seeing what was to come, we convinced ourselves that we stood apart, alone and exceptional. However, like the best politician or the worst chess player, we can change our minds. Nature is a web of relationships and, like it or not, we are included — if she will have us back.

HOW TO MAKE A FOOD CHAIN

Imagine you are sitting alone, in dappled light, beneath a tree on the side of a meadow. It's a wonderfully sunny day; a cow wanders into the meadow. If you are a carnivore, your focus locks onto the creature. You slowly realign your posture; your haunches flood with adrenaline and you sprint, in a blur, across the meadow. You leap onto the cow's neck, using your claws to hold on and your fangs to slice through a vulnerable artery. In a moment, it's over and you drag the carcass away for a blow-out meal. Carnivores are rare and rather solitary creatures. They are the last link at one end of what is called a 'food chain'. The other end is always plants.

Without plants, you wouldn't be here and neither would the carnivore. Plants live at the delicate interface between earth and sky. They are rooted in the moisture and minerals of the earth, but they reach for the sun, performing a near-miraculous feat of energy conversion in their process of photosynthesis. They use this captured energy to fund all of life's diversity. No other life form can do this; no other can be the first link in the food chain.

Your broad meadow is home to trillions of bacteria, millions of insects, hundreds of birds, rodents and scavengers. There will be herbivores of various sizes, the largest being that cow. Each of these species will eat and be eaten in a network of relationships made from lots of short food chains. In your meadow, peer closely at the underside of a leaf and you will see tiny insects. They are aphids and they are sucking the sap out of the plant. But then, along comes a ladybird. You needn't watch but the ladybird is going to eat the aphid. Across the meadow, a tree frog will catch sight of the ladybird and have it for dinner. A squirrel might have the tree frog for breakfast; later, a heron might eat the squirrel.

That's how a food chain works. Most chains involve, at most, four or five life forms. But, and this is so important, each life form is part of more than one food chain — that ladybird might have been eaten by a swallow instead of a tree frog. Their story starts at the same place, but now it's another story, another food chain. A similar process continues in the adjacent woodland, but with different species. The meadow and the woodland are habitats and because they are near to one another there will be a few food chains that knit the edges of these habitats together. The process is similar in the aquatic world, where plants such as single-celled algae float in the water and capture the sun's energy before they are harvested by water-dwelling creatures.

This chain-making goes on and on, the whole world over. As the chains crisscross each other and knit habitats together, they make the worldwide food web: an astonishing and complex assembly of life forms and living processes. If one life form is removed, all others must adjust; they turn to one of the other food chains of which they are a part. If two life forms, or three or perhaps a whole habitat is removed, this leads to loss of diversity, and diversity, as so beautifully expressed by natural historian Edward O. Wilson, is 'the property that makes resilience possible'. It is fair to say that resilience equates to survival. If diversity is reduced, survival is less likely.

Imagine you are sitting beneath the tree again. The cow wanders into the meadow to graze. You marvel at its size and wonder how the creature can be so large and powerful when all it eats is grass. The cow is a 'primary consumer' in the food chain. As a herbivore, it eats only plants and derives all of its nutritional needs from them. The carnivore can't do that. It still *needs* the nutrients the plant world provides, but it can only *get* them by eating a herbivore or an omnivore. The carnivore is an 'indirect consumer', who nevertheless remains totally reliant on plants.

Carnivores such as eagles and tigers are 'apex predators'; they have to eat flesh to survive. An entire habitat and all the life forms in it must sponsor the apex predator's solitary place at the far end of the food chain. If their habitat is altered, they are often the first species to disappear because they do not have other options. Most humans are not carnivores, but omnivores: deriving the nutrients they need from either the flesh and fluids of an animal, or directly from plants. This means you have a choice. Unfortunately, folk can get caught up in a pretence, believing humans are meant, or have a right, to be apex predators. To continue this self-deception, we must see the living world as a resource solely for our use. We must stand outside the web of life and believe that it is *for* us, but does not pertain to us. We must convince ourselves that we are essential and dominant, but that our errors do not matter. We must accept the impossibility of feeding all members of our own species and the inequalities that result.

Currently, collectively, we are undermining natural systems by dismantling food chains, habitats and whole ecosystems. Natural systems are being replaced with intensive livestock farming and monoculture crops. Neither of these link to any natural food chain, or foster diversity of species. Both are implicated in gross misuse of land and water, soil loss, pollution, climate change, and cannot, ultimately, meet the nutritional needs of the world's growing population. In adopting a plant-based diet, you become a 'primary consumer', deriving all that you need directly from the plants you eat. In doing so, if we all act quickly, you become part of a solution, too.

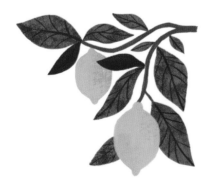

LIFE AND THE COLOUR GREEN

Life exists because plants harness the energy of sunlight. This should be headline news. There should be thousands of 'OMG!' texts sent at dawn every morning. We need reminding of this magnificent, breathtaking fact: the plant world enables and supports us entirely. But for plants and the processes they promote, none of us would be here.

For the past three billion years, the 'engine' for life has been pigments held within plant cells. These pigments are the chlorophylls (a and b), which let you see the plant's colour as green; and the carotenoids, which let you see the yellow to orange colour of a plant. Carotenoids protect chlorophyll from being damaged by excess light. They are present in green plants throughout the seasons, but chlorophyll hides their colours. In a woodland, for instance, carotenoids become apparent when the chlorophylls start to break down prior to leaf fall, causing the beautiful autumn (fall) display of orange and yellow leaves. Plant pigments become energized when they absorb the wavelengths of visible light, namely sunlight. When energized, chemical reactions occur that enable the plant to combine water and carbon dioxide to form carbohydrates for growth and storage. This process is called photosynthesis: the use of light (photo) to manufacture (synthesise).

The chlorophyll molecule is nearly identical to the haemoglobin molecule in your own red blood cells. Both molecules are pigments, but, while chlorophyll holds magnesium at its centre, haemoglobin holds iron. Chlorophyll transports energy from the sun; haemoglobin transports oxygen from the air you breathe. What a team! In your body, chlorophyll promotes healing and minimizes inflammation and infection. It stimulates enzymes that produce vitamins K and E. The accessory pigment, carotene (a carotenoid), is also known as pro-vitamin A because it is converted to vitamin A in your liver. These crucial nutrients, and many others as well, are available from eating green, leafy vegetables and the yellow/orange 'carotene' foods such as squash, carrots, pumpkins and cantaloupe.

Plant life is a complex and highly organized life form with tens of thousands of unique species. The resources a plant requires for its existence are sunlight, water, carbon dioxide and the minerals and nutrients it can obtain from the soil. A plant does not need to chase after its next meal. It thrives and feeds the world of animals and humans in stillness, taking only these ingredients into itself. Give me a kitchen door that opens onto a garden, a field, or any piece of land that can entice even a single plant to grow. For one plant, its roots clinging to what it has found for itself, can tell us more about the whole world than we can discover through long years of theoretical studies. Today I planted a pot of parsley; tomorrow I will plant a tree.

DEEP ECOLOGY

In 1962, biologist Rachel Carson's book *Silent Spring* exposed the devastation chemicals wreak on the natural world. Her book alerted populations around the world of the long-term dangers of misuse of chemicals, and she is often called the mother of the modern ecology movement. Her assertion that we humans exist 'as part of a vast web of life, all of which needs to be taken into account' struck a chord with many. In 1969, poet and ecology theorist Gary Snyder wrote an essay entitled *Four Changes*, which focused the movement that had grown up in the years following publication of Carson's book by laying out in clear terms a 'deep ecology' position. He suggested an adjustment in thinking that would allow a new human identity to emerge. Specifically, that a 'revolution in consciousness' would 'create an awareness of "self" which includes the social and natural environment'.

In its broadest definition, deep ecology is an understanding of interconnectedness that invites you to act with reverence and care toward the whole of life. It recommends that you reconsider your relationship with other life forms as well as your treatment of them. It urges against the view that humans — and their needs and desires — are more important than other aspects of the living world (anthropocentrism) and suggests that you value all of life, the whole of Nature, as one integrated system of which you are but one part. If you were able to roll back the scroll of history and listen to the insights of earlier people who, like yourself, have been made alert, you would hear the same message repeated: 'Take care! We humans are only one part of this whole, living world.'

Our ancestors knew this because they lived it. They subsisted by fitting in with the life patterns around them. Then, from approximately 10,000 BCE, a new way of living was gradually established. Humans began to form settlements, cultivate crops and domesticate animals. This period is sometimes referred to as the Neolithic Revolution. Later, in the early eighteenth century, came the Industrial Revolution, which saw rural populations leave their gardens and orchards, and migrate to cities for the promise of a better life. Finally, from the 1930s through the postwar years, more huge changes in agricultural, medical and scientific practices again altered the way people related to the land. The promise of 'better living through chemistry' convinced whole populations that they not only could, but also had a right to conquer microbes, insects, weeds and Nature herself. What was touted as an era of invincibility was, beneath the gleam of modernity, the infancy of environmental disaster. These revolutions, though millennia apart, mark degrees of 'drift' in the relationship between humans, their food and the living planet.

Deep ecology asks that you do not act to establish dominance and control over Nature, nor arrogantly, wastefully or destructively 'spend' natural resources, nor pit yourself in opposition to Nature. Rather, it invites you to reidentify; to see humans as one species in union with the whole.

ON A KNIFE EDGE

When you are trying to balance, bare-footed, on the sharp edge of a knife, a reasonable question to ask is, 'How long is the blade?' or perhaps, 'How deep will it cut?' A recent paper from the Alliance of World Scientists makes a clear declaration that 'planet Earth is facing a climate emergency'. The paper is signed by more than 13,600 scientists from 156 countries and suggests six 'critical and interrelated' measures that *everyone* can take to reduce the effects of the emergency. At a time when the global environmental crisis is ignored by many and denied by some, and when there are clear efforts to confuse or disempower the urgency of the message, this report is clarifying and oddly calming. The latter because it gives straightforward guidance for urgent action. In other words, it measures the blade, leaving no doubt about the potential severity of the wound.

The six steps suggested, summarised here, encompass the key issues that underpin climate change. They are:

* Energy: stop using fossil fuels and replace with clean, safe, low-carbon renewables
* Short-lived pollutants: promptly reduce emissions of: black carbon from diesel engines, wood-burning stoves, forest fires; hydrofluorocarbons (HFCs) used in refrigeration and air-conditioning units; methane from intensive farming of cows, sheep, goats and buffalo
* Nature: protect and restore forests and ecosystems, curtail loss of habitats and of species diversity
* Economy: stop overexploitation of ecosystems and resources in favour of long-term sustainability
* Population: stabilize or reduce growth, strengthen human rights and ensure universal education
* Food: reduce the consumption of animals (especially ruminants) and animal products by eating mostly plant-based foods

BUTTERFLY POWER

What a bullet-point list cannot do is adequately expose the interrelated nature of these key issues. You will likely have heard of the 'butterfly effect,' a phrase now used in common parlance but originally part of an academic inquiry into predictability by Edward Lorenz, a Professor of Meteorology at MIT. In his 1972 paper, he asked, 'Does the flap of a butterfly's wings in Brazil set off a tornado in Texas?' Apparently, yes, it can. Small differences introduced into living or dynamic systems can initiate significant and even unexpected outcomes. The mechanism for this is interrelatedness, though often of a scale and type that we humans do not yet fully understand.

So, though we might sit at our kitchen tables and pity ourselves for living in what could be the end times for humankind, in fact, we would do better to think of ourselves as butterflies. Each one of us can 'flap our wings' to influence the outcome of this crisis.

Though we are encouraged to think of ourselves as powerless, our individual choices — what we buy, what we eat, how and where we travel — are already proven to be powerful. Our choices, and those of generations before us, have brought us to this moment and this situation. Our job, now, is to make new choices that will allow our children, and our biosphere, a future.

Here is a To Do list to show how individuals can make a difference:

* Use the 80/20 rule (page 9) to steer yourself and family toward a plant-based diet.
* Waste not, want not: globally, approximately one-third of food is wasted in production phases, or through consumer practices, leading to poor nutrition, loss of income and hunger. To minimize waste, reduce the amount you buy, use it before its expiry date, donate to food banks and come up with ideas to help solve this problem.
* If you have outdoor space, begin to garden it with food plants and/or plants that support a diverse range of wildlife, including bees, birds, insects, toads, frogs, and small, vulnerable species such as Britain's hedgehogs.
* Take an allotment or join a community garden scheme.
* Learn about compost and build a compost heap for family use.
* Plant trees. Aim to plant one tree each year for each member of your family. Include food trees, such as fruit and nut species, as well as long-lived species native to your region.
* Become aware of wild or semi-wild habitats in your area and learn how you can support them.
* Assess your use of short-term pollutants (above) and act to minimize your reliance on them.
* Assess and reduce your use of household chemicals that might pollute land and water systems.
* Recycle everything you can; aim to create a zero-waste household.
* Involve your children in what you do so they gain skills and broaden their awareness.

Do what you can in your own home and locale. You can't do it all and you can't do it alone. But that's the whole point!

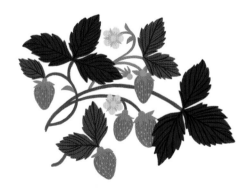

EVERY NOTE'S A VOTE

One note of your cash could be the one that saves the world: every purchase you make is a vote cast in favour of the product you buy and the companies and practices associated with it. It's not always easy to see the realities of a purchase because they often are not obvious. In fact, sometimes they are downright hidden from you. 'Hidden' suits many; there are people who earn a lot of money by keeping information away from inquisitive minds. They earn that money from you, through your purchases, at the same time as they keep you in the dark. This describes a form of moral impoverishment that is not doing any of us any good. At base, it describes a world where people don't care for each other, don't care for the planet and don't care about what or who comes next. So, go ahead and make a fuss. You are more powerful than you think! Use your daily purchases to help nudge businesses, corporations and governments back into line. It's your world as much as theirs. You can make your moral preferences heard by speaking the language they listen to: money.

Switching to veganism affects how and where you spend your money and is a tremendously powerful vote for change; one that can help to mitigate climate change crises. Happily, food producers are listening and responding – now more than ever. They continually monitor spending and, seeing the surging trend toward plant-based diets, are striving to remain in your favour by changing what they produce and how they produce it. They are getting the message – it's ringing loud and clear through all those cash registers. You might not be in a position to campaign, write letters or research the working conditions in your ex-favourite fast-food joint. But you can still think before, during and after any purchase you make.

Here are a few simple questions that can help you to reorganize the way you spend your money. For any product, ask yourself:

1 Who benefits?
2 Who or what is harmed?
   * Is it the environment, by way of habitat destruction, waste and pollution?
   * Is it the workers who have, perhaps, been exploited, underpaid or imperilled?
   * Is it animals, through exploitation, suffering and cruelty, illness and death?
   * Is it the consumer by being sold unethical, unhealthy or unsafe products?
3 What is it made of?
4 How is it made?
5 How is it made available?
   * Does its packaging cause destruction?
   * Does the advertising used to sell it cause harm?
   * Is it sold in a truthful and responsible manner?

Most people make purchases every day. It makes sense to use these as opportunities to send a message; to cast your vote and transform the act of spending into an act of care and consideration.

BOUNDARIES AND RIGHTS

Human and animal rights are all about boundaries: where you draw them, why you draw them and how you enforce or protect them. With boundaries, you can say 'Only what is inside the boundary is correct' and 'Anyone outside the boundary is a waste of space', or even 'Failure to be my gender, background, income band or nationality means you are outside the boundary of my awareness and I do not acknowledge you.' Like borders, the lines we draw can structure identities and systems that enrich us – or they can destroy, causing dislocation from others and from a broader, more generous way of being.

It's true that not all boundary lines are chosen; a significant number are imposed by culture, tradition or the legal system. It was not so long ago that in the United Kingdom and other places around the world women could not vote and homosexuality was illegal. Deep, prolonged misery and conflict result from such lines because they serve only a very few and demean or impoverish the rest. Of course, there are some lines that are clearly beneficial, including those that protect children, preserve privacy or engender respect. Personal boundaries are also crucial to maturation, autonomy and self-esteem. Perhaps the knack in drawing boundary lines is to think carefully and ask many questions before we commit. Because such lines can either highlight and support our qualities, or they can imprison and diminish us.

Rights are boundaries intended to enhance the lives of those who have them. They are entitlements that define how you may act as well as how others may act upon you. Crucially:

* You *have* rights, just by being in the world.
* You may *claim* rights by choosing or asserting them.
* You might be *given* rights because others determine that you deserve them.
* Rights always need to be *protected*.
* Rights are *distributed*, sometimes naturally and with compassion, but most often using governments and laws and assessments of status.

SENTIENCE AND SUFFERING

Historically, when distributing rights, an assessment of status would include species, gender, wealth and occupation. A more modern measure of status is sentience: the capacity to perceive through use of the senses, and to have an inner experience as a consequence. Often, the allocation of rights balances precariously on this assessment – after all, if you aren't sentient, why bother giving you rights?

Uh-oh. Some problems here. How do you *know* if another being can sense and feel? You could ask them, but what if they are a baby? What if they don't speak the language? What if they have been injured and cannot signal their understanding? What if they are an animal? You might observe them and judge whether they can see, hear, smell, taste and touch. But how do you know if they are feeling; if their sensory experience also creates an inner experience?

One way is to discern whether they can suffer. Suffering can be defined, in part, by what it isn't. It isn't joy or playfulness. It isn't calm or pleasure or confidence. Suffering is the opposite of those and includes inner states such as loneliness, anxiety and fear, as well as outer displays of suffering such as crying, rage, pain or panic. Suffering can arise from within or it can be inflicted. So, by observing the baby, the foreign-speaker, the injured being and the animal, we can see that they all suffer and therefore must be sentient. They all pass the assessment of status, and rights may be distributed to them.

ANIMALS HAVE RIGHTS TOO

As animals are sentient, then they, like humans, have natural rights: those that exist just by being born. They include the right to life; the right not to be killed; the right to live in the society of its species. These rights exist whether or not a law is in place to protect or enforce them. But animals cannot claim their rights. In practical, human-centric terms, that means animals do not have rights except those they are given by human intervention. Therefore, the onus is on people to acknowledge the natural rights of animals and to protect those rights on behalf of the animal.

Historically, as a collective, humans have drawn a boundary around themselves that denies other animals any relevance beyond their use to humans. Some religions have condoned this by asserting that humans have been given dominion over the Earth and everything that lives upon it. Capitalism encourages it by selective allocation of value to the Earth, its resources and its living populations. The modern scourge of narcissism – the 'it's all about me' affliction – represents this boundary, too; but drawn so tightly that it fits only one person. But we can't have it both ways. On the one hand, as *Homo narcissus*, demanding all the attention, all the prizes, all the Earth's bounty and resources; on the other hand, eagerly seeking meaning and connection with nature, each other and with life itself.

The current state of the environment and the plight of wild and livestock animals are symptoms of boundary lines that are inappropriate and no longer tenable. But we can change them. As we feel ourselves becoming ever more isolated within our strangulating boundaries, more spiritually impoverished and destructive, perhaps we can, instead, begin to acknowledge and protect the rights of other species as, in a similar way, we do for babies and those humans unable to claim theirs for themselves.

SPECIES-ISM AND THE GOLDEN RULE

You will have heard it many times. It rolls off the tongue, along the lines of: 'Treat others as you would like them to treat you.' It is so simple and sensible – a place in your heart knows this is the correct way to behave. But how well this 'golden rule' works depends on how you define 'others'.

In 1970, an English philosopher named Richard Ryder created the word 'species-ism' to name the prejudice that excludes non-human animals from the care and protection that humans try to give to other humans. A 'Declaration against Species-ism' was composed in 1977 at a gathering of academics discussing animal rights, held at Cambridge University. In an interview discussion held in 2013, Ryder said: 'The point I was trying to make is that we are all related. All species are related biologically and through evolution. And instead of treating the other species like objects, we should be treating them like evolutionary cousins …'

Australian philosopher Peter Singer carried the idea – and the word – forward to wider public attention when he introduced his 'principle of equal consideration'. It states that when you act for your own interests, you should also place equal importance on how your actions affect the interests of others. This sounds remarkably like the golden rule, but what upset many people was that this consideration might be applied to animals when, for most of history, humans have exploited other creatures and excluded them from the sphere of human care. Nevertheless, Ryder and Singer continued to question the relationship humans have with animals. A comparison they used to illuminate the status quo was the experience of discrimination against other humans on the basis of sex and race.

You know how this works already. A person who treats a member of the opposite sex as being of less value than a member of their own sex is considered to be sexist. A person who treats a member of a different race as being of less value than members of their own race is considered to be racist. A person afflicted with these states of mind is not considering what the 'different' or 'opposite' person feels or needs. Instead, they are giving priority to the needs and feelings of their own race and sex: favouring it, making it more relevant, more important, more correct or deserving. This is prejudice, whereby the status or wellbeing of the other is disregarded and devalued in an unreasoning way. Removing reason from behaviour is chilling because behaviours then become open to malevolence and a clear intention to do harm. Prejudice rarely stops at sex and race. It appears to be a condition of extreme fear, expressed in a hybridized form of anger, which is directed at anyone or anything that presents with differences. Unfortunately, a person who is prejudiced in this way is often profoundly intractable; unable or unwilling to see or to remedy their affliction.

Both Ryder and Singer knew they had a hard nut to crack. Yet the comparison they made with sexism and racism successfully brought the discussion to a wider audience. Singer added a clarifying point, a sort of leveller, by bringing up the matter of pain. He suggested that having a capacity to feel pain is necessary to having *any* 'interests' and, as both human and non-human animals *do* feel pain, both have interests in preventing it. Applying his golden rule, his 'principle of equal consideration', Singer said that a reasoning person would not assign more importance to the pain of a human than to the pain of another species of animal. To do so would be to act in the manner of a sexist or racist: but this time as a species-ist.

Many objections have been raised to the idea of giving equal consideration to non-human creatures. A long list of 'what humans can do that animals cannot' has been drawn, presumably to show that because animals do not have language, for instance, they are of less value than humans. There does not, however, appear to be a list of what animals can do that humans cannot. Having language or other attributes of being human does not make it acceptable to be prejudiced. It should make it less acceptable; yet there are still more prejudices lurking in the shadows of this discussion. For instance, consider the fact that some humans are less intelligent than some animals. Such humans might be mentally handicapped or simply infants: not yet developed. Should these people be deprived of their 'interests' because they are not as capable as other humans? Should they be treated as non-human animals currently are treated?

Until very recently, species-ism has been the norm. Holding up a mirror to human prejudice has caused distress and embarrassment to many. But it has also shown that, although we have a long way to go, we can apply the 'golden rule' and learn to correct assumptions and behaviours that demean us all.

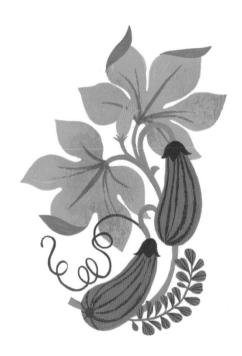

DOGS AND CATS GO VEGAN

People who wouldn't usually give a moment's thought to 'rights' can suddenly become adamant supporters of animal rights when the subject of vegan pets is raised. The reaction goes something like this: 'It's okay for humans to go vegan, but it's unfair to impose a plant-based diet on animals!' The topic is a contentious one, without doubt, and it is often asserted that it's hypocritical for vegans to have pets. It's true, there is much that is wrong about pet ownership: the animal is controlled, confined, sometimes exploited by being made to work and generally is prevented from living naturally and autonomously. Even the most well-meaning human is caught in an overtly hierarchical relationship with the animal, including the responsibility of feeding it.

But humans have lived communally to mutual benefit with dogs for approximately 30,000 years and with cats for about 10,000 years. Being vegan does not bar that relationship. In general, vegans don't usually buy a pet; they instead make a home for a companion animal brought from a rescue centre, so the animal is not euthanized or used in laboratory experiments.

For many people, vegan or not, opening a can of indefinable meat in smelly gravy is a really big call, especially if it is likely to harm the companion animal. And it does harm them; you could be feeding your companion animal the diseased body parts of other animals, including of their own species, unwittingly turning it into a diseased cannibal. Buying meat-based pet food is buying into the entire flesh, egg and dairy industries, with all the ethical, environmental and health issues that involves.

But, back to rights: it's not about the human; it's about the animal. What would be best for their needs? In fact, what are their needs? Dogs are formally classified as carnivores, but are biologically omnivorous. In the course of their domestication, they adapted and can now produce more starch-digesting enzymes than true carnivores. Cats on the other hand are true carnivores. They do not derive adequate nutrients from a diet rich in carbohydrates. They require a high intake of protein such as is naturally present in meat. If meat is not part of their diet, they require supplements to provide necessary nutrients. Just like humans, both dogs and cats are prone to serious disorders if adequate nutrients are not provided.

It is, however, possible to provide all the nutrients an animal needs using plant-based ingredients.

* Combine either pre-formulated or homemade plant-based foods with supplements to achieve an optimal nutrient profile without using animal ingredients. See Resources for suppliers and recipe providers.
* Ensure the diet product contains all the nutrients essential to the animal's needs. A veterinary nutritionist can help you to design the best meal plan for your pet.
* A transition period is usually necessary, allowing your pet time to accept the new diet. For instance, mix 10% of new food with 90% of established food, gradually altering the ratios until 100% new food is achieved. The 80/20 rule again!

FEASTS AND CELEBRATIONS

JERUSALEM ARTICHOKE SOUP
WITH TRUFFLE OIL

Jerusalem artichokes look rather unpromising, but their flavour is unique. They're quick and easy to cook, as well as inexpensive, versatile and nutritious. The truffle oil is a treat but perfectly complements the flavour of the artichokes. Maybe because they both grow underground? I like to serve this soup alongside a stack of sandwiches, including Kohlrabi and Cucumber Sandwich (page 123) and Egg Salad Lookalike Sandwich (page 99).

SERVES 4

PREPARATION TIME 30 MINUTES

+ STANDING

300g (10½oz) Jerusalem artichokes

2 tablespoons untoasted sesame oil

2 large onions, finely chopped

¼ teaspoon black pepper

¼ teaspoon Chinese five-spice

1 litre (35fl oz/4 cups) vegetable stock or water

¼ teaspoon ground turmeric

Truffle oil, to serve

OPTIONS AND VARIATIONS

Use ¼ teaspoon ground cinnamon instead of the five-spice powder.

Scrub and rinse the artichokes, put them in a bowl and pour fresh water over them. Leave to stand for 5 minutes, then carefully lift them out. Scrub and rinse them again, then slice into small rounds.

Pour the oil into a saucepan set over a medium heat. Add the artichokes and onions, cover the pan and sauté for 15 minutes, stirring often. The vegetables should become very tender and start to caramelize.

Add the black pepper and five-spice powder, and cook for about 2 minutes.

Pour the stock into the pan, stir well and purée with a hand-held blender. Add the ground turmeric and stir well. Add another 250ml (9fl oz/1 cup) stock or water for a thinner texture, if preferred.

Bring the soup to a low simmer, then remove from the heat. Cover and set aside for an hour or so to allow the flavours to blend.

Reheat before serving. Ladle into bowls and lightly drizzle truffle oil over each bowful just before bringing to the table.

EXTREMELY OLIVE PIZZA

I like to use Kalamata olives here: they are large, dark and fleshy, and absolutely make this stripped-down, high-intensity pizza. I buy them from a grocer specializing in Middle Eastern foods, who ladles them, brine and all, into a jar for me. Call in some helping hands to make the preparation swift. Eating it takes no time at all. Keep it simple, and serve with Quickly Salad (page 93) or Entirely Green Salad (page 92).

MAKES 2 × 30cm (12in) PIZZAS

PREPARATION TIME 1 HOUR

1 quantity Rich Tomato Sauce (page 252)

1 quantity Easy Pizza Base (page 124)

500g (1lb 2 oz/1¾ cups) whole Kalamata olives (this weight includes their pits)

A little oil for greasing the baking sheets

OPTIONS AND VARIATIONS

Use other types of olive, if you wish – but Kalamata olives have the most intense flavour and cook well.

Prepare the sauce and the pizza base dough.

Invite friends or family members to come and help remove the olive pits and slice the olives in half. Pour the remaining olive brine into the sauce and stir well. (There is usually 3–4 tablespoons brine, which will be dark from the olive juices and salty, too.)

Preheat the oven to 200°C (400°F), and lightly oil two baking sheets.

Divide the pizza dough in half. Carefully press and spread a portion of dough evenly onto each of the baking sheets. Cover the pizza bases with the tomato sauce – use a bit more than you might think necessary, as it will dry out during the baking process.

Share the prepared olives between the two pizzas. Your aim is to cover the entire surface of each pizza with olives, right up close to the edges and with little space between them. Press them into the sauce as you place them.

Bake in the hot oven for 15–20 minutes until the edges of the crust are browned and crisp, then slice and serve.

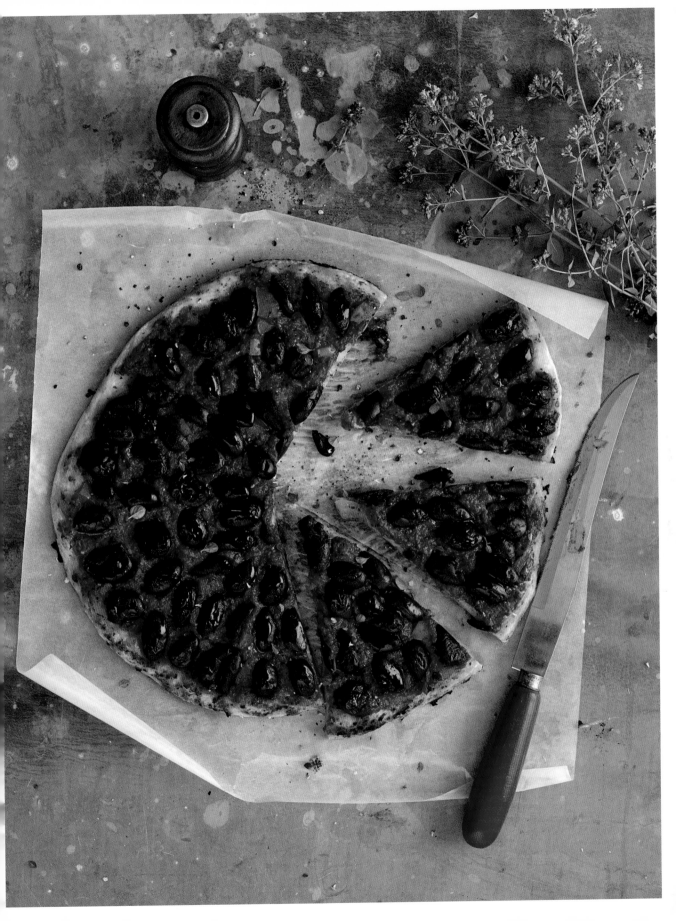

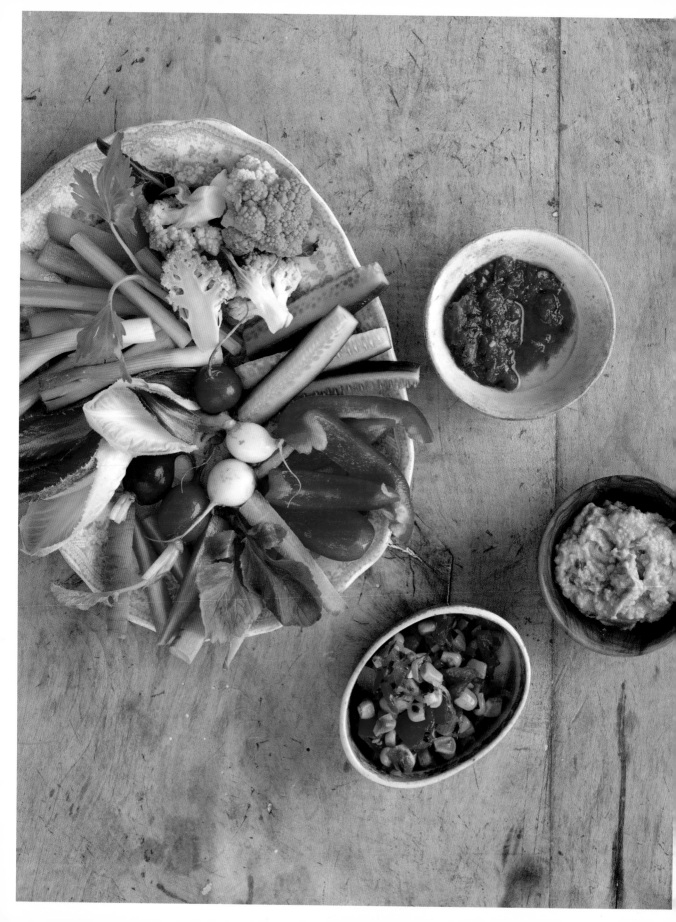

CRUDITÉS PLATTER

This is a surprise favourite with young people. The trick is to make it look so appealing that they forget they're eating healthy, raw fruit and veg. Provide individual plates and put a serving spoon in each dip.

SERVES 4–8

PREPARATION TIME 15 MINUTES

Choose a variety of fruit and vegetables from the list below, and make three or four of your favourite dips. Chill the dips while you prepare the fruit and vegetables, as suggested.

Pick one or two large platters, and arrange the crudités so they look irresistible. It's a matter of celebrating contrasts in texture and colour.

Put your selection of dips in small bowls, arrange them around the platters of crudités and see what happens!

VEGETABLES CRUDITÉS

Sticks of raw celery, carrot and courgette (zucchini), trimmed and cut to similar length

Cauliflower florets, trimmed to bite-size

Turnip and kohlrabi, cut into 'chips'

Sweet peppers (capsicums), all colours, cut into sturdy strips that will support a dollop of dip

Chicory leaves, trimmed at the bottom end

Spring onions (scallions), trimmed

Cucumber, cut into sticks or thick coins

Radishes, washed and the tap root trimmed away, but not the green 'handle'

Baby cos (romaine) lettuce, leaves separated and trimmed at the bottom

Sprouted mung beans, in a bowl with kitchen tongs to serve

FRUIT CRUDITÉS

Apples, cut into eighths or sixteenths, and tossed in lemon juice to prevent them from turning brown

Oranges, broken into segments

Grapes, all colours – delicious for dipping!

Tomatoes, quartered if they are large; otherwise use whole cherry tomatoes

Bananas – leave the peel on, but slice each banana into five or six chunks; each chunk keeps its 'wrap' and therefore its colour until it is peeled and eaten

Nectarines, sliced

Whole cherries

DIPS

Great Guacamole (page 73)

Margarita Yogurt Dip (page 90)

Red Pepper and Tomato Salsa (page 133)

Adzuki Bean Ragout (page 133)

All-Day Chutney (page 247)

Sweetcorn and Pepper Relish (page 134)

Tahini Lemon Whip (page 83)

Herb and Onion Bean Butter (page 71)

Mung Bean Pâté (page 77) can be added, but would need a knife to spread it into a celery stick, for instance

BERRY-MARINATED TEMPEH ROAST

This dish takes a little time to prepare, but it's worth it for the visual appeal and the all-round specialness of it. Adding tamari just before serving beautifully brings together the sweetness of the berries and earthiness of the tempeh – so don't be tempted to leave it out. Trust me! This is delicious with Entirely Green Salad (page 92) and a slice of Rosemary Twist (page 164) to dip into the juices, or alongside Seaweed and Potato Cutlets (page 206) and Warm Broccoli Salad (page 151).

SERVES 4

PREPARATION TIME 45 MINUTES

+ 4 HOURS MARINATING

4 tablespoons untoasted sesame oil

400g (14oz) tempeh, sliced into discs, wedges or rectangles no more than 1cm (½in) thick

250g (9oz) fresh raspberries

125g (4½oz) fresh blueberries

Juice of 1 lemon

4 teaspoons tamari

OPTIONS AND VARIATIONS

Adjust the ratio of raspberries to blueberries to suit availability and your personal preference.

Heat half of the oil in a large frying pan (skillet) and add the tempeh slices, allowing room for them to be moved and turned. Cover the pan, and sauté the tempeh over a medium heat for 10 minutes on each side, adding more oil if needed.

Meanwhile, mix together the berries and lemon juice in a bowl. Use a fork to slightly crush some of the berries, but be sure to leave some of them whole.

Select a serving dish (a heatproof one if you plan to serve this warm), and spread half the berry mixture in the bottom of it. Arrange the cooked tempeh slices over the berry mixture, and spoon the remaining berries on top. Cover the dish and leave to marinate in the refrigerator for at least 4 hours (but no more than 12), turning the tempeh pieces now and then during that time.

Just before serving, tilt the serving dish to collect a spoonful of marinade. Pour this over the top of the tempeh and put a few of the whole berries on top as well.

Serve immediately or, if you want to serve it warm, put the dish under a hot grill (broiler) to heat through for about 5 minutes.

The final touch: sprinkle a teaspoon of tamari over each serving.

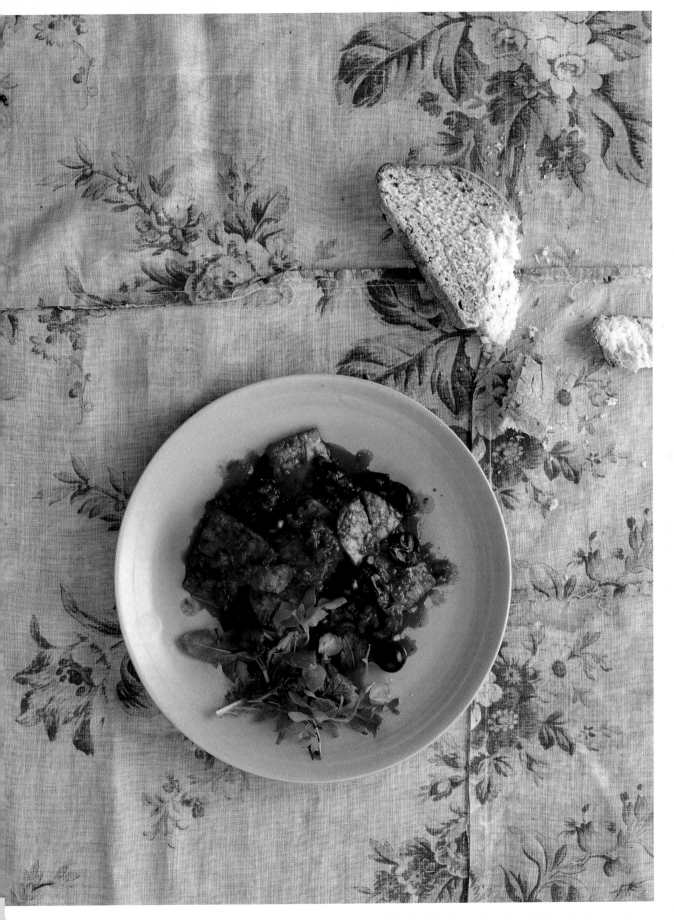

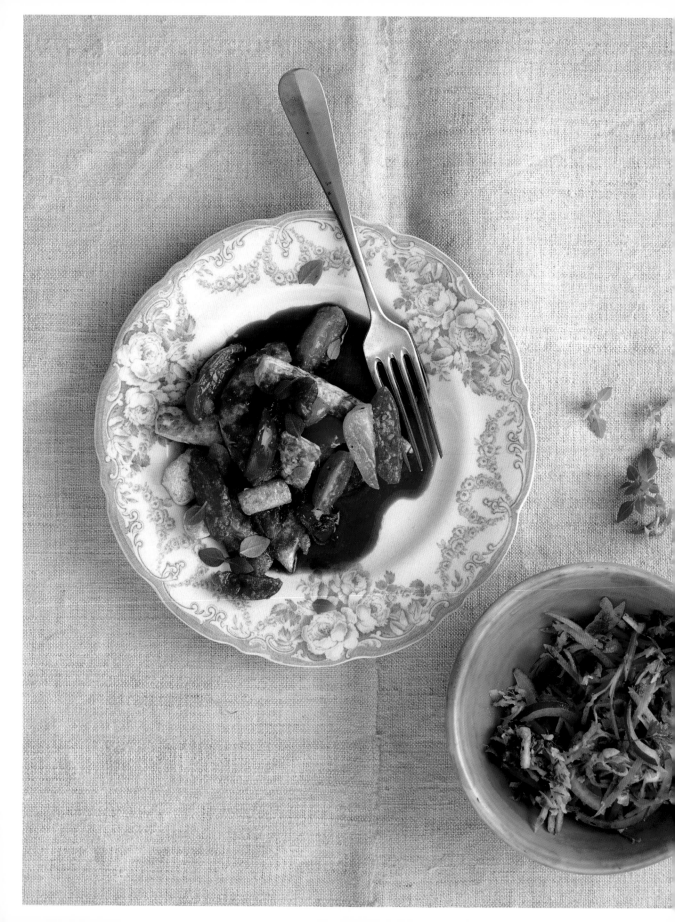

MARINATED TOFU AND TOMATO PLATTER

These tofu slices go very quickly – I often double the recipe. I prepare this when I'm in the kitchen anyway and have a bit of time for the marinade to work before guests arrive for a buffet lunch. The garlic and tomatoes add flavour to the dish, as well as colour and texture. This is popular alongside a portion of Great Grated Salad (page 192) or Rice, Radish and Spice Salad (page 90).

SERVES 4

PREPARATION TIME 1 HOURS

+ 3-4 HOURS CHILLING

4 tablespoons untoasted sesame oil

400g (14oz) firm tofu, drained and cut into strips 1cm (½in) thick

6 garlic cloves, sliced

6 cherry tomatoes, quartered

FOR THE MARINADE

100ml (3½fl oz/scant ½ cup) tamari

100ml (3½fl oz/scant ½ cup) apple cider vinegar

Juice of 1 lemon

2 tablespoons grated fresh ginger

Pour half of the oil into a large frying pan (skillet), and arrange the tofu strips to fit. Cover the pan and set over a low to medium heat. Fry the tofu for 10–12 minutes, then turn and cook on the other side, adding 1 tablespoon more of the oil if needed.

While the strips are cooking, prepare the marinade. Mix together the ingredients in a jug (large measuring cup). Set aside until needed.

When the tofu strips are lightly golden on both sides, arrange them in a pretty serving dish in a single layer.

Pour the jug of marinade into the frying pan, and return the pan to the heat for 2–3 minutes. Pour the hot marinade over the tofu slices.

Add the remaining 1 tablespoon oil to the frying pan. Once heated, add the garlic and cherry tomatoes. Cover the pan, increase the heat to medium and cook for 5 minutes. Spoon the cooked garlic and tomato, along with any pan juices, over the marinating tofu slices.

Set the dish aside to cool, then cover and chill for 3–4 hours. Jostle the dish once or twice during this time, to ensure that the marinade is well distributed. Serve.

CABBAGE AND PINK SALAD

Shreds of beetroot (beets) bring a beautiful pink colour to this dish that is gradually taken on by the other ingredients. Pink peppercorns and red onion add more pink, as well as their own flavour hits, both of which are gently contrasted by cooling cucumber. This salad suits all seasons, and looks stunning beside Tofu and Couscous Magic (page 126) or Egg Salad Lookalike Sandwich (page 99).

Mix together the cabbage, onion, cucumber and salt in a large bowl. Use wooden spoons or your hands to lightly squeeze the ingredients together in a kneading motion for 1–2 minutes, to soften the vegetables and release some of their juices. Leave the mixture for 10 minutes, stirring or kneading once or twice more in that time.

Tilt the bowl and tip away any liquid that has been released by the vegetables. Stir in the grated beetroot, pink pepper and Velvet Vinaigrette, and serve.

SERVES 4

PREPARATION TIME 30 MINUTES

750ml (26fl oz/3 cups) finely shredded white cabbage

1 small red onion, finely sliced

1 small (12cm/4½in) cucumber, thinly sliced

1 tablespoon sea salt

1 small beetroot (beet), grated

A little ground pink peppercorn

Velvet Vinaigrette (see right)

OPTIONS AND VARIATIONS

Use a sweet white onion instead of the red onion. It will take on the pink colouring, but contribute a more mellow onion flavour.

VELVET VINAIGRETTE It is worth keeping a jar of this in the refrigerator – it seems to go with almost everything – but let it warm to room temperature before serving so that the olive oil returns to its liquid state. Measure 60ml (2fl oz/¼ cup) apple cider vinegar (or the same quantity of lemon juice) into a clean jam jar or similar (make sure it has a tight-fitting lid). Add a large pinch of salt and mix with a fork. Add 2 teaspoons each of Dijon and wholegrain mustard, and 2 small crushed garlic cloves, and stir again. Pour in 120ml (4fl oz/½ cup) extra virgin olive oil, put the lid on the jar and shake briskly to blend. Serve immediately or chill until ready for use. Wonderful on Dressed Greens and Beans (page 154), Entirely Green Salad (page 92) or freshly steamed Brussels sprouts.

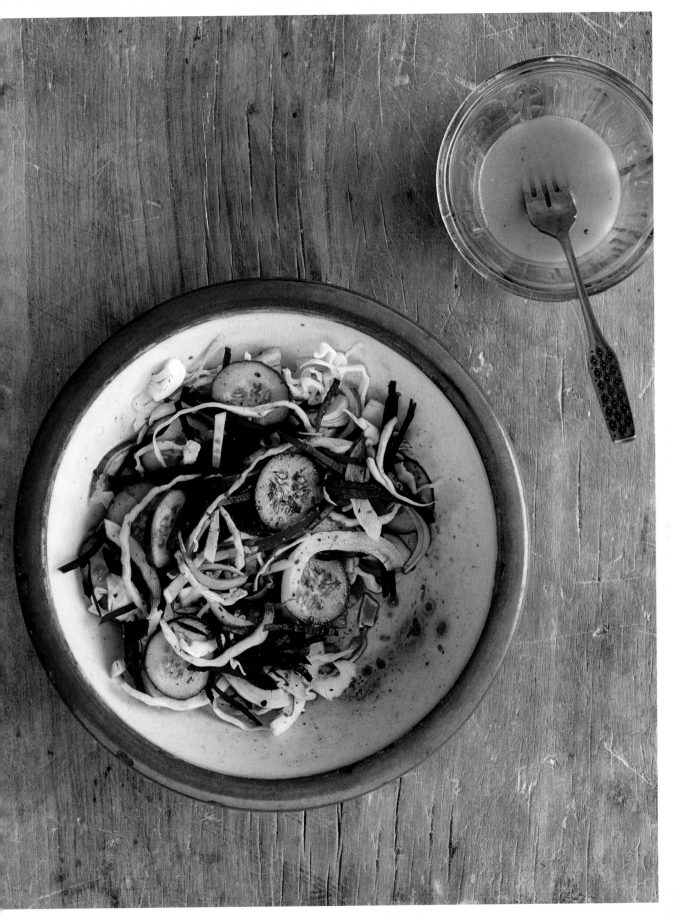

HOT PEANUT SAUCE

The peanut is another food that originated in South America and has travelled the globe, settling anywhere it can enjoy a long, warm growing season. Peanuts are an extraordinary food with a unique flavour. They are a powerhouse of nutrients, with more than 300 derivative products, including oil and flour. Sometimes known as groundnuts, they are a natural emulsifier, so this sauce can be as thick or thin as you wish. It is so delicious you will want it poured over everything at first! Try it over Chunky Tofu in Greens (page 117), Beansprout and Noodle Chaos (page 196) or Stir-fried Vegetables over Spiced Noodles (page 114).

Pour the oil into a saucepan. Add the garlic, chilli and ginger, and sauté over a low heat for 10 minutes. Stir once or twice. Add the chopped tomato and cook for a further 5 minutes, stirring often.

Add the peanut butter to the saucepan, and stir to blend with the other ingredients. Gradually add half of the lime juice and all of the tamari, and continue stirring.

Add more lime juice, a little at a time, as the sauce thickens. Keep stirring and adding lime juice as needed, to achieve the consistency you prefer. Remove from the heat and serve hot.

MAKES ABOUT 250ml (1 CUP)

PREPARATION TIME 30 MINUTES

2 teaspoons groundnut (peanut) oil (I use the oil that sits on top of the peanut butter in a newly opened jar)

6 garlic cloves, crushed or finely chopped

1 fresh red or green chilli, deseeded and finely chopped

1 tablespoon grated fresh ginger

1 large tomato, finely chopped

4 tablespoons peanut butter

Juice of 4 limes (about 140ml/4½fl oz)

2 tablespoons tamari

OPTIONS AND VARIATIONS

Use ½ teaspoon dried chilli flakes instead of the fresh chilli. For an added tangy depth, stir in 1 tablespoon date or pomegranate molasses when adding the lime juice to adjust the consistency.

NATURAL THICKENERS A few foods act to thicken any liquid to which they are added:

* Fresh ginger will slightly thicken the sauce produced while stir-frying vegetables
* Turmeric will thicken a soup, sauce or dhal, as well as add colour to it
* A spoonful of peanut butter will thicken a sauce if it is added during cooking
* Tahini will mix with a liquid such as lemon juice or water to create a thick, fluffy texture
* Mustard, either dry or prepared, will help two liquids come together to make a sauce or dressing

ALL-DAY CHUTNEY

I make this slow-cooked chutney when I'm busy in the kitchen anyway, such as during the routine that follows the weekly visit to the farmers' market. Though the chutney takes a few hours to cook, it requires only a little attention during that time. Meanwhile, it fills the kitchen with wonderful aroma and makes enough to put aside a jar or two for the weeks ahead. It can make a nice gift for a friend. It's spicy, so a little goes a long way. Try a spoonful with Simple Red Lentil Dhal (page 201), Kohlrabi and Cucumber Sandwich (page 123) or Three-Grain Risotto (page 184).

MAKES 1.5 LITRES (6 CUPS)

PREPARATION TIME 3 HOURS

500ml (17fl oz/2 cups) apple cider vinegar

250g (9oz) soft light brown sugar

2 onions, finely chopped

1 whole garlic bulb, cloves separated and chopped

2–4 fresh chillies (to taste), finely chopped

80g (2¾oz) piece of fresh ginger, finely chopped or grated

6 medium apples, peeled, cored and diced

250g (9oz) dried fruits, such as raisins, sultanas (golden raisins), currants or goji berries, or a mixture

1 small cauliflower, florets quartered

2 teaspoons mustard seeds

1 teaspoon ground turmeric

½ teaspoon ground cinnamon

OPTIONS AND VARIATIONS

Add 1 large chopped beetroot (beet) for a darker colour and a hint of earthy flavour.

Pour the vinegar and sugar into a large nonreactive saucepan. Set it over a medium heat, and stir well to dissolve the sugar.

Add the remaining ingredients and stir well. Cover the pan, reduce the heat and cook, stirring occasionally, for at least 2 hours. Aim for a thick, textured and spicy chutney.

Gather together the jars you want to use and arrange them, and their corresponding lids, in a roasting pan or large cake pan. Boil the kettle and fill the jars and the insides of the lids with boiling water. Set aside until the chutney is ready.

When the chutney is cooked, empty the hot water from the jars and immediately fill them with the hot chutney. Empty the water from the lids, and put them on the jars immediately to create a strong seal. Leave to cool.

This chutney will keep for 4–6 weeks if the sterilizing instructions on page 43 are followed.

RUBY ROOT SOUP

I first made this for my family's arrival home, cold and tired, after a long journey through chilling weather: now, I can only think of it as a winter meal. There are delicious 'hidden' ingredients that give extra body and texture to this soup, leaving the beetroot to make its big ruby-red statement. Serve this soup beside a wedge of Mung Bean Pâté (page 77) and a slice of Splendid Wholesome Loaf (page 120). A spoonful of Creamy Onion Sauce (page 115) swirled into each bowlful creates a stunning garnish.

SERVES 4

PREPARATION TIME 1 HOUR

1 medium beetroot (beet)

2 tablespoons untoasted sesame oil

1 large onion, chopped

2 celery stalks, finely chopped

1 medium carrot, chopped

1 medium parsnip, chopped

1 medium potato, chopped

1 teaspoon vegan bouillon powder

1 teaspoon dried basil

½ teaspoon dried thyme

½ teaspoon black pepper

¼ teaspoon ground cloves

Salt, to taste

OPTIONS AND VARIATIONS

Use dried oregano instead of the thyme, and ground allspice instead of the ground cloves. If you prefer a thinner soup, add 250ml (9fl oz/1 cup) additional water.

Steam the beetroot over a medium heat for about 30 minutes until tender. Meanwhile, prepare the other ingredients.

Pour the oil into a large saucepan, and add the onion, celery, carrot, parsnip and potato. Cook over a medium heat for 15 minutes, stirring occasionally.

Lift the beetroot from the steaming basket, and use a fork to steady it on the chopping board while you trim away the taproot and leaf stems. Scrape away and discard the skin, then chop the beetroot.

Add the beetroot to the other vegetables along with the bouillon, herbs and spices. Continue cooking for a further 10–12 minutes until the vegetables are tender. Stir occasionally.

Once the roots are tender, add 1 litre (35fl oz/4 cups) water. Purée the ingredients using a hand-held blender, taste and adjust the seasonings, and bring to a low simmer before serving.

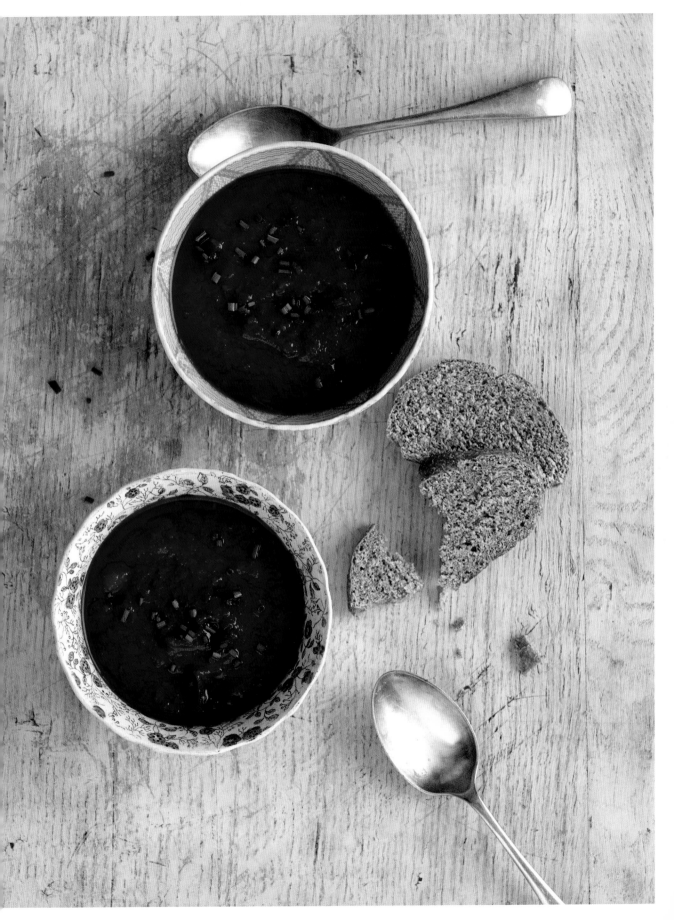

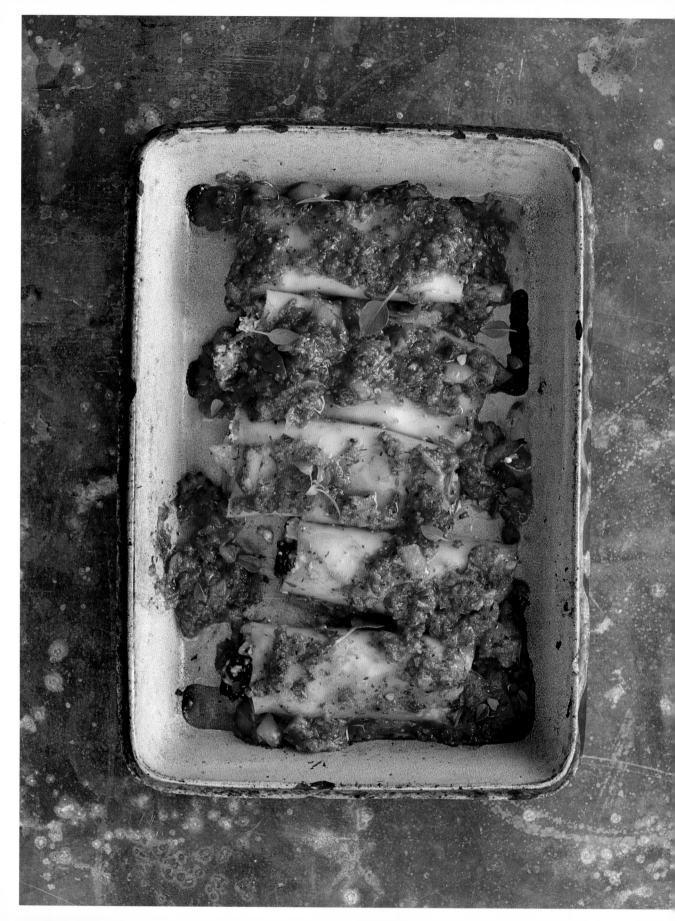

HERB AND TOFU CANNELLONI

I always feel like I'm back in kindergarten when I make this dish: it's great fun, but I still make a mess. I've heard that some people actually roll their own cannelloni, something I have not yet tried. When I take this out of the oven, I prefer to let the dish sit for a few minutes before serving. The sauce and filling both hold their heat and benefit, in flavour and texture, from a little cooling. I like to serve this with Broccoli Almond Sizzle (page 190) or a simple Entirely Green Salad (page 92).

Select an ovenproof dish that will hold all the cannelloni tubes, approximately 23cm × 30cm (9 ×10in). Preheat the oven to 200°C (400°F), and lightly oil the dish.

Heat the 1 tablespoon oil in a saucepan, and cook the leek, onion and garlic, covered, for 10 minutes over a medium heat, stirring occasionally. Add the parsley, dried basil and olives. Stir over the heat for 2–3 minutes, then cover the pan and remove from the heat.

In a separate bowl, gently stir together the tofu and 200g (7oz/2 cups) of the vegan cheese. Add the onion and herb mixture; stir well but gently, so as to retain some texture.

Use a teaspoon to fill the cannelloni with the tofu mixture, arranging the stuffed tubes in the ovenproof dish as you go. Cover the filled cannelloni with the Rich Tomato Sauce and bake in the oven for 30–35 minutes.

Reduce the oven temperature to 180°C (350°F). Sprinkle the fresh basil and the remaining vegan cheese over the hot cannelloni and return to the oven for 5 minutes. Serve.

SERVES 4

PREPARATION TIME 1¼ HOURS

1 tablespoon untoasted sesame oil, plus extra for oiling the dish

1 small, tender leek, finely chopped

1 small onion, finely chopped

8 garlic cloves, finely chopped

100g (3½oz/3⅓ cups) finely chopped fresh flat-leaf parsley

1 teaspoon dried basil

160g (5¾oz/scant 1 cup) olives, pitted and sliced

400g (14oz) firm tofu, drained and finely cubed (about 2¼ cups prepared)

300g (10½oz/about 3 cups) grated Cheddar-type vegan cheese)

250g (9oz) dried cannelloni

1 quantity Rich Tomato Sauce (page 252)

140ml (4½fl oz/generous ½ cup) chopped fresh basil

OPTIONS AND VARIATIONS

Use a mozzarella-type vegan cheese, instead of a Cheddar-type.

SUPERB LASAGNE

The first time I served this, my family dubbed it 'superb lasagne' and asked me not to make it more than once a year for fear of overindulgence! Serve with Quickly Salad (page 93) and a small portion of Fresh Borlotti Bean Salad (page 104). You might need to slightly adjust the quantity of lasagne sheets, depending on the shape and size of your baking dish.

SERVES 4

PREPARATION TIME 1 HOUR

Oil for greasing the ovenproof dish

1 quantity Rich Tomato Sauce (opposite)

About 900g (2lb) dried lasagne sheets

400g (14oz) firm tofu, drained

400g (14oz) fresh baby spinach, washed and drained

250g (9oz) vegan Cheddar-type or mozzarella-type cheese, grated

165g (5¾oz) sun-dried tomato and black olive tapenade

OPTIONS AND VARIATIONS

Add 1 medium courgette (zucchini), finely chopped, before the final layer of lasagne.

Preheat the oven to 250°C (500°F), and lightly oil a deep 3-litre (100fl oz/12-cup) ovenproof dish. Ladle about 200ml (7fl oz/scant 1 cup) of the tomato sauce into the dish, and spread over the bottom to make an even layer.

Arrange a layer of lasagne sheets over the sauce, breaking them to fit as necessary. Crumble the tofu and distribute it evenly over the layer of lasagne. Distribute one-third of the spinach over the tofu. Next, ladle another 200ml (7fl oz/scant 1 cup) of the tomato sauce over the spinach.

Add a second layer of lasagne sheets and press them down. Distribute one half of the remaining spinach over the lasagne sheets. Sprinkle half of the grated cheese evenly over the layer of spinach. Ladle another 200ml (7fl oz/scant 1 cup) of tomato sauce over the layer of cheese.

Add a third layer of lasagne sheets and press them down. Distribute the remaining spinach over the lasagne. Ladle another 200ml (7fl oz/scant 1 cup) of tomato sauce over the layer of spinach.

Add a final layer of lasagne sheets. Spread the tapenade onto the lasagne sheets. Ladle over the remaining sauce, ensuring that the edges of the lasagne sheets are covered. Bake in the oven for 10 minutes, then reduce the temperature to 180°C (350°F) and bake for about 30 minutes more.

Test to see whether the pasta is cooked by inserting a sharp knife through the layers in the centre of the dish. When the lasagne sheets are tender, sprinkle the remaining cheese over the top. Return the dish to the oven for about 5 minutes, to melt the cheese.

The lasagne will 'set' and slice more easily if left to cool for a few minutes before serving. Be careful – it retains heat!

RICH TOMATO SAUCE

This is a versatile, deeply flavoured sauce. Ladle it over a plate of spaghetti, or use it to make Simple Herb and Caper Pizza (page 125) or Superb Lasagne (opposite). Cook it in an enamel or stainless-steel pan, not a cast-iron one, so that the sauce doesn't take up the taste of iron.

MAKES ABOUT 1 LITRE (4 CUPS)

PREPARATION TIME 20 MINUTES

1 tablespoon untoasted sesame oil

1 whole garlic bulb, cloves separated and chopped

1 medium onion, finely chopped

1 fresh chilli (red or green), finely chopped

1 sweet pepper (capsicum) (red, yellow or green), diced

1 tablespoon dried basil

1 teaspoon dried oregano

1 litre (35fl oz/4 cups) tomato passata (purée)

OPTIONS AND VARIATIONS

Use ¼ – ½ teaspoon dried chilli flakes, to taste, instead of the fresh chilli. For a more textured sauce, add 2–3 chopped fresh tomatoes after softening the vegetables. Cook until tender before adding the herbs and passata. Use Your Own Tomato Compote (page 254) in place of the passata.

Measure the oil into a frying pan (skillet), and sauté the garlic, onion, chilli and sweet pepper over a medium heat, stirring once or twice.

Cook the vegetables for about 10 minutes until they are very tender. Add the chopped fresh tomatoes at this point, if you choose that option. Finally, add the dried herbs and the passata. Stir well and simmer over a low heat for about 20 minutes while you ready the rest of the meal.

If a smooth texture is preferred, you can purée the sauce using a liquidizer or hand-held blender.

YOUR OWN TOMATO COMPOTE

When neighbours, friends and family are all begging you to take the extra tomatoes they've grown, make this simple, useful sauce and store a few jars in the back of the cupboard. You'll need a Mouli (rotary hand mill) and some preserving (canning) jars. The tomato flavour is intense and a real joy to work with. Use the compote as a base for soups or sauces – just add spices, herbs, and sautéed garlic, onions or sweet peppers (capsicums). Try it in place of the passata in Rich Tomato Sauce (page 253) or with your favourite additions on Simple Herb and Caper Pizza (page 125).

MAKES A LOT

PREPARATION TIME 4–6 HOURS

Large quantities of fresh tomatoes

Salt, to taste

OPTIONS AND VARIATIONS

Include 2 apples, cored and quartered, when cooking the tomatoes. They will add sweetness and body to the compote without overwhelming the tomato flavour.

Wash the tomatoes, cut them in half and add them to your largest pan, including any juices that escape when you slice them.

Cover the pan, set it over a medium heat and cook until the tomatoes are soft and easily lose their form when pressed with a wooden spoon. This shouldn't take long, especially if you stir them from time to time

Pass the cooked tomatoes through the medium milling plate of a Mouli, discarding the skins and residue left behind in the funnel.

Return the tomato sauce to the pan and bring to a low simmer. Leave it to cook, uncovered, over a low heat, to reduce by one quarter to a third of its original volume. Reducing evaporates some of the water and intensifies the natural sweetness and flavour of the tomatoes. Stir occasionally. Once the sauce has reduced and reached a consistency you're happy with, add some salt to taste.

To prepare your storage jars, put them in a large baking pan and pour boiling water into and over them, including their lids and seals. (Let others know that the jars are hot.) Tip out the hot water from the jars just before you're ready to fill them with compote.

Ladle the hot compote into the jars, filling them to within 3cm (1¼in) of the top. Fasten the lids while everything is still hot, and set aside to cool. Your jars of tomato compote will keep, unopened, for a month or two if stored in a cool, dark place.

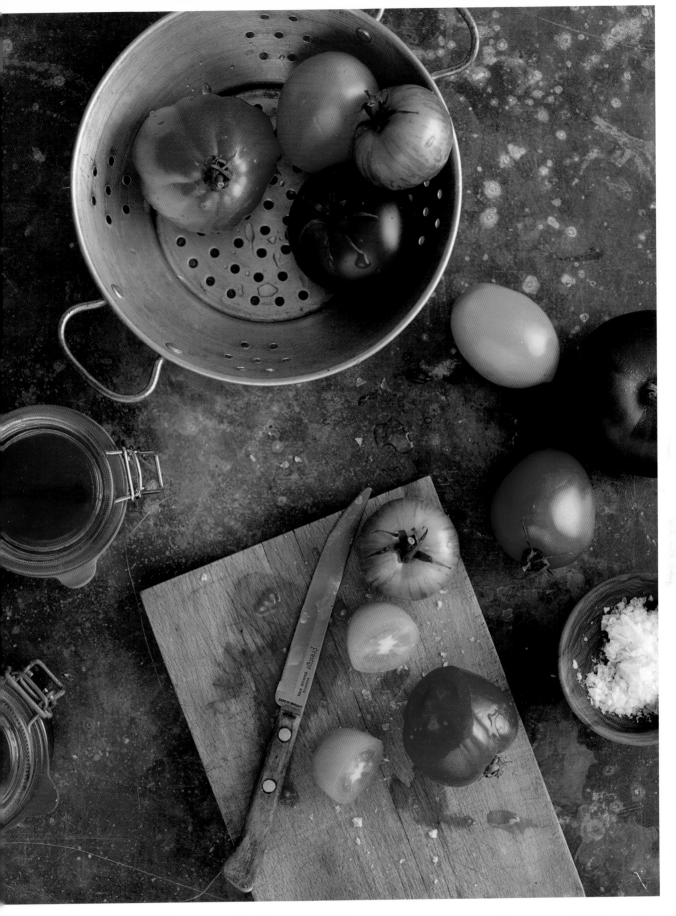

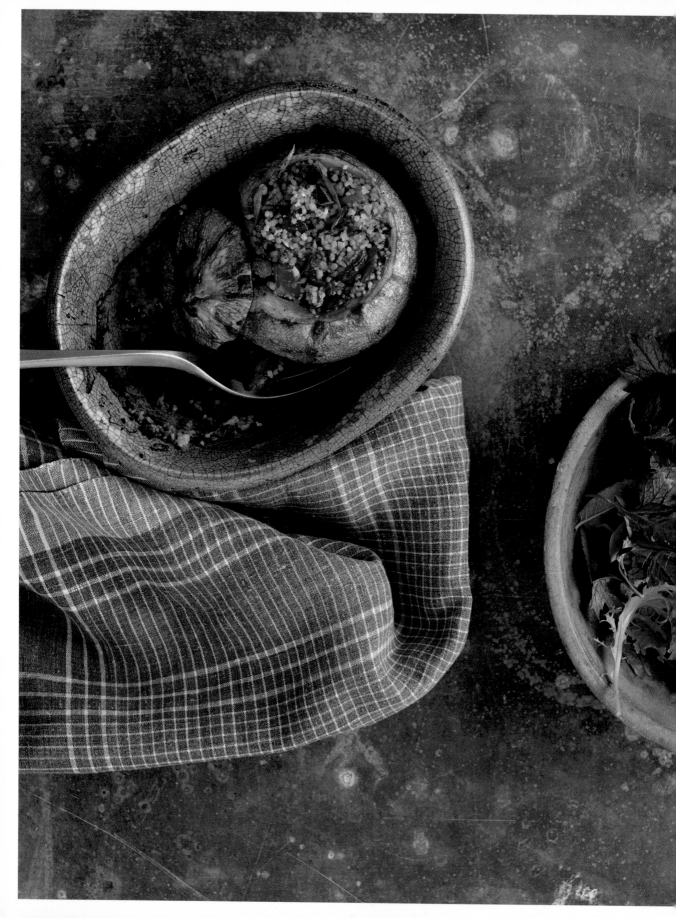

STUFFED PUMPKIN BAKE

All pumpkins are not equal! I recommend those with dark orange flesh because, usually, they are packed with flavour and have a dense texture. These baked pumpkins hold their heat, so it's fine to bring them out of the oven and let them cool a little before serving. The pumpkins can be broken apart or carefully 'mined' for a little tender pumpkin flesh along with each spoonful of filling. Serve with All-Day Chutney (page 247). If you can't find little pumpkins, use two larger ones: simply slice them in half, deseed and fill the halves, serving one half to each person.

SERVES 4

PREPARATION TIME 1 HOUR

4 small pumpkins, each roughly 10cm (4in) in diameter

200g (7oz) soft tofu, cut into small cubes

100g (3½oz/½ cup) couscous

50g (1¾oz) crushed walnuts

1 medium red onion, finely chopped

20g (¾oz/⅔ cup) finely chopped fresh flat-leaf parsley

2 medium tomatoes, finely chopped and juices retained

1 teaspoon dried basil

½ teaspoon dried oregano

½ teaspoon black pepper

¼ teaspoon Chinese five-spice

OPTIONS AND VARIATIONS

Use pine nuts or roughly crushed hazelnuts instead of walnuts.

Preheat the oven to 200°C (400°F), and pour cold water to a depth of 1cm (½in) into one large or two medium lidded ovenproof dishes.

Now make a 'lid' to each pumpkin by carefully slicing off its top, cutting about a quarter of the way down its height. Use a metal spoon to scrape out the seed pulp from inside the lid and body of each pumpkin. Discard or compost the seed pulp. Set aside each pumpkin and its lid.

Mix together the remaining ingredients in a bowl, slightly mashing the tofu as you stir. Divide this mixture evenly among the four pumpkins and press the filling down inside each one.

Pour 2 tablespoons cold water into each pumpkin. Place the 'lid' on each pumpkin or put them in the dish beside the pumpkins. Cover the ovenproof dish, and bake in the oven for 15 minutes. Reduce the oven temperature to 180°C (350°F), and cook a further 30 minutes.

Carefully lift the pumpkins from the dish using a broad spatula. Top with their 'lids' and serve.

✳ **STEAMED PUMPKIN** Pumpkins tend to cook quickly and you can often get two meals out of a medium-sized one. An easy way to prepare them is to steam them. Cut a pumpkin in half, top to bottom, and scoop out the seed pulp. Slice these halves again, into two or four pieces, and put these segments, skin side up, in a steaming basket set over simmering water. Steam for 15 minutes and serve hot or cold. Use any leftover portions to make Pumpkin and Parsnip Soup (page 203).

SPINACH AND ARTICHOKE TART

This savoury tart is easy to make at any time of year. It can be eaten hot or cold, and is one of those dishes that most people will recognize, so it is a good one to serve to guests. Excellent served with Tempeh Crisps in Pomegranate Glaze (page 167) and Quickly Salad (page 93).

MAKES 1 LARGE TART

PREPARATION TIME 1 HOUR

½ quantity Vegan Shortcrust Pastry (page 265)

1 medium potato, thinly sliced

½ teaspoon black pepper

100g (3½oz/2 cups) spinach, finely chopped

½ teaspoon Chinese five-spice

8 canned or preserved artichoke hearts, chopped or sliced

1 medium tomato, chopped

400g (14oz) firm tofu

250ml (9fl oz/1 cup) soya milk

1 teaspoon dried basil

½ teaspoon dried oregano

½ teaspoon ground turmeric

OPTIONS AND VARIATIONS

Add 2 tablespoons nutritional yeast flakes to the custard sauce as you blend it.

Preheat the oven to 200°C (400°F), and line a 28cm (11¼in) pie dish with the prepared pastry.

Arrange the potato slices on the pastry base, and sprinkle with the black pepper. Next, press the spinach in a layer over the potatoes. Sprinkle the five-spice powder over the spinach, and scatter the artichokes and tomato on top.

Blend the tofu, soya milk, herbs and turmeric in a blender, or in a mixing bowl using a hand-held blender, until smooth. Slowly pour the custard over the ingredients in the pie dish, spreading it evenly to the edges of the tart.

Bake in the oven for 10 minutes, then reduce the temperature to 180°C (350°F) and cook for 35–40 minutes.

Cool for 5 minutes before serving hot, or leave to cool completely.

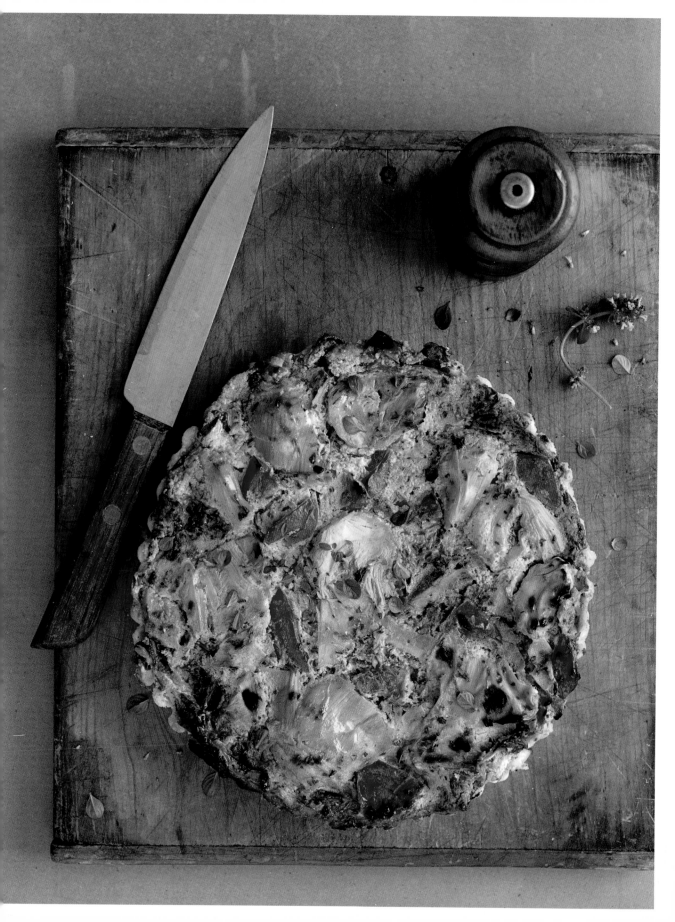

PRETTY GOOD PUNCH

It's a good feeling to provide a special, refreshing drink that goes well with a long Sunday lunch or an evening meal on the patio. It's free from alcohol, so you can happily share it with young people. But, if you prefer, add a chilled bottle of Sauternes or 200ml (7fl oz/scant 1 cup) rum. Serve with Epic Cubes (page 81) or just plain ice in each glass.

SERVES 4

PREPARATION TIME 30 MINUTES

+ CHILLING

2 teaspoons green tea (in a tea ball) or 2 teabags green tea

4 whole cloves

6cm (2½in) piece of cinnamon stick

1 lemon

1 lime

1 orange

100ml (3½fl oz/scant ½ cup) elderflower cordial

OPTIONS AND VARIATIONS

Use ginger cordial instead of the elderflower. Add a sprig of fresh lemon balm or garden mint to the mixture before chilling.

Pour 1 litre (35fl oz/4 cups) boiling water over the green tea leaves or teabags. Leave to brew for 3 minutes, then remove the tea ball or teabags, and add the cloves and cinnamon stick to the hot liquid. Cover and set aside to cool.

Halve the lemon, lime and orange. Squeeze the juice from one of the halves of each fruit and pour into a large measuring jug (large measuring cup). Stir in the elderflower cordial. Add the cooled and strained green tea, stirring well.

Slice the remaining citrus halves, and layer the slices in a large jug (pitcher) or punch bowl. Pour over the mix of tea, citrus juices and elderflower cordial. Add the cinnamon stick and fresh herbs if you wish. Chill and stir gently before serving.

FAMILY HISTORY FRUITCAKE

Favourite recipes often develop over time according to the preferences of family members: a new ingredient here, an altered method there. This one has evolved over four recent generations, so far, but is likely to have started much earlier, in unwritten versions. Legend tells of an aged aunt who liked to pour a small glass of brandy over her portion! Save a little of the icing to spread across cut surfaces, to keep the cake moist between servings.

MAKES 1 LARGE FRUITCAKE

PREPARATION TIME 4 HOURS

+ 3 WEEKS MATURING

300g (10½oz/1½ cups) soft light brown sugar

200g (7oz) vegan margarine, melted, plus extra for greasing

150ml (5fl oz) tahini

Juice of 3 lemons

450g (1lb/3 cups) plain (all-purpose) flour

450g (1lb) dried currants

450g (1lb) sultanas (golden raisins)

450g (1lb) raisins

200g (7oz) candied citrus peel

70g (2½oz) dried or glacé cherries

100g (3½oz/1 cup) flaked almonds

1 teaspoon each of ground cinnamon, ground ginger and ground nutmeg

2 tablespoons barley malt syrup or blackstrap molasses

2 tablespoons apple cider vinegar

TO DECORATE THE CAKE

170g (6oz) favourite jam (jelly)

500g (1lb 2 oz) marzipan

100g (3oz) vegan margarine

300g (10½oz/2½ cups) icing (confectioners') sugar, plus extra for rolling the marzipan

1 teaspoon vanilla or almond extract

Preheat the oven to 150°C (300°F), and lightly oil a 23 × 30cm (9 × 12in) deep cake pan.

Blend together the sugar and margarine in a large bowl. Add the tahini and lemon juice, and blend well.

In a separate bowl, stir together the flour, dried fruits, candied peel, almonds and spices.

Mix together the syrup and vinegar in a jug (large measuring cup). Stir this mixture into the other wet ingredients, and whisk together.

Blend the wet and dry mixtures together in the large bowl. Tip the batter into the prepared cake pan, and press it firmly and evenly into the pan.

Bake in the oven for 2–3 hours until risen and brown, and a skewer or the tip of a sharp knife inserted into the centre comes out clean.

Leave the cake to cool in its pan on a wire rack. Keep the cake in its pan, cover the top with a clean cloth and set it aside (where no one will find it!) for three weeks, to allow the flavours to mature.

After three weeks, place the cake upside down on a cake board covered with baking paper. Spread a thin layer of jam over the sides and top.

Dust your work surface and rolling pin with a little icing sugar, and roll the marzipan into a thin sheet, large enough to cover the sides and top of the cake. Carefully lift the marzipan and position it onto the cake. Gently press the marzipan onto the cake – you will feel it stick to the coating of jam. Trim away any excess marzipan around the bottom of the cake.

Prepare the icing. Put the margarine in a bowl and add the icing sugar, a little at a time, stirring after each addition until it is well blended. Add the vanilla extract last of all, and spread the icing over the marzipan. Leave to stand for at least 1 hour before serving.

CHOCOLATE, ORANGE AND ALMOND CAKE

Looking for an immersive chocolate experience? This is my go-to cake for birthdays and those cherished once-in-a-while treats and celebrations.

MAKES 1 SANDWICH CAKE

PREPARATION TIME 1 HOUR

350ml (12fl oz/1½ cups) almond milk

1 tablespoon apple cider vinegar

100ml (3½fl oz/scant ½ cup) oil

100ml (3½fl oz/scant ½ cup) tahini

100ml (3½fl oz/scant ½ cup) freshly squeezed orange juice

350g (12oz/2⅓ cups) plain (all-purpose) or wholemeal (whole-wheat) flour

150g (5½oz/⅔ cup) granulated sugar

100g ground almonds

60g (2¼oz/½ cup) dairy-free unsweetened cocoa powder

1 tablespoon orange zest

2 teaspoons bicarbonate of soda (baking soda)

1 teaspoon baking powder

FOR THE CHOCOLATE ICING

250g (9oz) good-quality dark chocolate

70g (2½oz) vegan margarine

300g (10½oz/2½ cups) icing (confectioners') sugar

1 tablespoon almond milk

1 teaspoon almond extract

OPTIONS AND VARIATIONS

Use a 23 × 30cm (9 × 12in) cake pan to make this a single-layer cake.

Preheat the oven to 200°C (400°F), and lightly oil two 20cm (8in) cake pans.

In a large bowl, stir together the almond milk and vinegar. Leave this mixture to stand. Blend the oil, tahini and orange juice together in a measuring jug (large measuring cup).

In a separate bowl, mix together the flour, sugar, almonds, cocoa powder, orange zest, bicarbonate of soda and baking powder.

Pour the blend of oil, tahini and orange juice into the bowl with the almond milk and vinegar mixture. Whisk these together.

Add the dry mixture to this wet mixture and stir well, but briefly.

Turn the batter into the prepared cake pans, and put them in the oven. Immediately reduce the oven temperature to 180°C (350°F), and bake for 25–30 minutes until risen and springy. A skewer or the tip of a sharp knife inserted into the centre should come out clean. Cool the cakes in the pans for 5 minutes, then transfer to a wire rack to cool completely before icing.

To make the icing, break the chocolate into a heatproof bowl set over a pan of simmering water. (Ideally, the bowl should not touch the water. However, not everyone is set up for that. Instead, if you have a metal or ceramic heat dispersing pad, such as comes with a pressure cooker, place that in the bottom of a saucepan and rest your heatproof bowl on it. Add water to the saucepan and bring it to a simmer over a low to medium heat.) Stir occasionally until the chocolate is melted. Add the margarine to the bowl and melt it in with the chocolate.

Remove the bowl from the heat and stir in the icing sugar, a little at a time. Add the almond milk and extract, and stir well.

Spread a thin layer of icing between the layers of cake, fit the cake together and spread the rest of the icing over the top and sides. Let the icing cool before serving.

✳ **CAROB** is a pod from a shrub or tree also known as the locust tree, or St John's bread. You can buy carob as a spread, a syrup or a powder, and use it instead of chocolate. Use the spread in sandwiches; the syrup to make a hot or cold 'chocolate' drink; and the powder to make a 'chocolate' cake. Carob has no caffeine, but it does have a high mineral content.

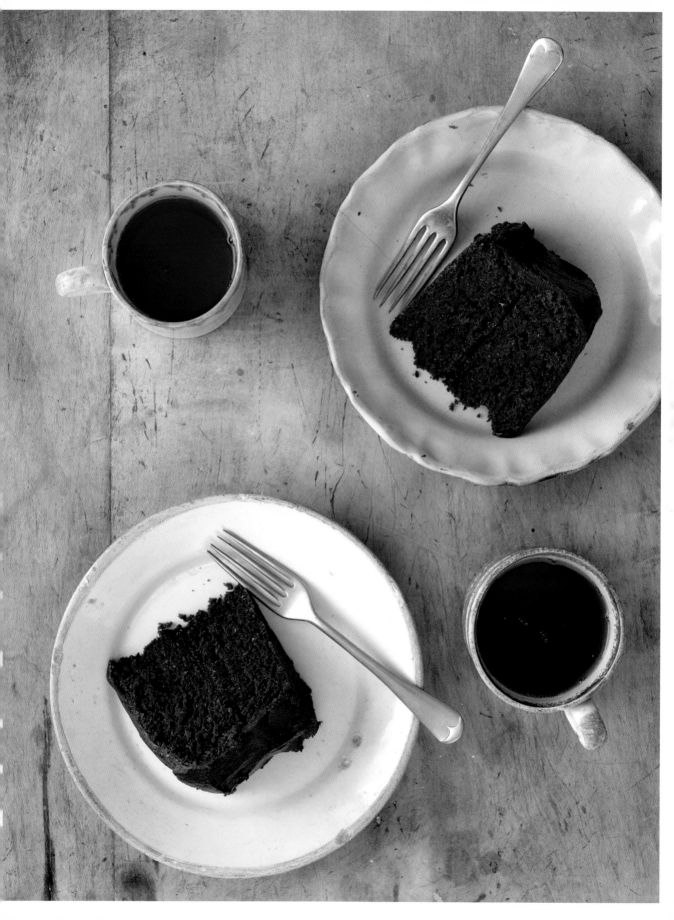

SWEET CRUMB CRUSTS

No rolling pin is required in the making of these crusts: simply press the chosen mixture into the baking dish. Each recipe makes one 28cm (11¼in) tart base crust.

COOL COCONUT CRUST This is used for a no-bake chilled pie. Heat 80g (2¾oz) coconut oil in a frying pan (skillet) over a low heat. Add 250g (9oz/3 cups) desiccated (shredded) coconut and cook, stirring often, for 7–10 minutes until lightly golden. Add 3 tablespoons plain (all-purpose) flour and continue to stir the mixture over the heat for a further 5 minutes. Press the mixture into a pie dish and chill for at least 1 hour. Add the filling and chill the finished pie.

SWEET PRESS PASTRY You can use this crust as a base for a chilled or cooked topping. Mix together 100g (3½oz/⅔ cup) plain (all-purpose) flour and 40g (1½oz/⅓ cup) icing (confectioners') sugar in a bowl, and rub 50g (1¾oz) vegan margarine or coconut oil into the mixture to make a fine crumb. Press into the pie dish and bake at 180°C (350°F) for 15 minutes.

BISCUIT CRUMBLE CRUST Melt 80g (2¾oz) coconut oil in a pan, and mix in 300g (10½oz/2¾ cups) finely crushed vegan digestive biscuits (graham crackers). Press into the bottom of the pie dish and up the sides. Bake for 10 minutes at 180°C (350°F), then cool and add the filling for a chilled pie.

VEGAN SHORTCRUST PASTRY

This makes a light, flaky crust for tarts and pies. For best results, chill the dough all day or overnight: it will get rather hard, but when you leave it at room temperature for 20–30 minutes it becomes ideal for rolling and shaping (however, if you let it sit out for too long, it is less easy to manipulate). Enjoy creating your own distinctive pie style with rolled or forked edges, decorative pastry appliqué, signature slice marks and sweet glazes.

ENOUGH FOR 2 TARTS OR 1 PIE

PREPARATION TIME 20 MINUTES + 1 HOUR CHILLING

150g (5½oz/1 cup) plain (all-purpose) white flour, plus extra for dusting

75g (2¾oz) coconut oil

50g (1¾oz/⅓ cup) fine cornmeal

Measure the flour into a large bowl. Add the coconut oil and 'cut' it into the flour, using a fork or table knife, to create an even texture throughout. Add the cornmeal, working it in the same way to create an even texture.

Add 100ml (3½fl oz/scant ½ cup) ice-cold water, and quickly work it into the dough with your fingertips. Shape the dough into a ball, cover the bowl and chill in the refrigerator for at least 1 hour, and up to 24 hours.

Remove the pastry from the refrigerator 20–30 minutes before use, and bring to room temperature. Lightly flour your work surface and a rolling pin. Keep a little extra flour to one side, to use as needed.

Divide the dough in two, and knead one portion on the work surface to ensure an even consistency. Roll out the pastry into a round or rectangle, as required, to a thickness of 5mm (¼in).

Lift the pastry into the pie dish and press into place, trimming off any excess. Roll the remaining pastry in the same way, to make the top crust, or to line a second pie dish.

✳ **READY-MADE PASTRY** You can buy vegan puff pastry in the chilled or frozen food sections of many supermarkets. It works well but, unfortunately, some brands are made with palm oil. Overuse of this oil is destroying the natural habitat of the world's remaining wild-living orangutan population. Please check the label. If you like this recipe above, store it in useful portion sizes in the refrigerator or freezer until you need it.

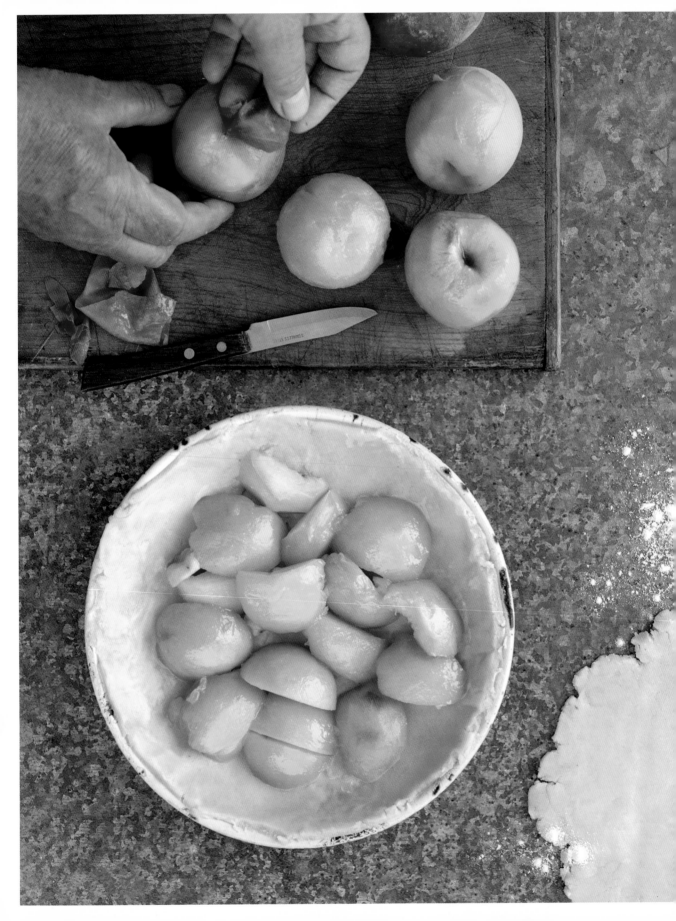

SWEET PIE COLLECTION

Here are four simple fruit pies to serve as snacks or desserts.

APPLE PIE Preheat the oven to 180°C (350°F). Line a 28cm (11¼in) pie dish with Vegan Shortcrust Pastry (page 265) and prepare the top crust. Mix 50g (1¾oz/¼ cup) soft light brown sugar and 25g (1oz/¼ cup) oat flakes (rolled oats) with ½ teaspoon each of ground cinnamon and ground cloves. Add 50g (1¾oz/½ cup) flaked almonds, and mix well. Distribute half of this mixture onto the pastry base and top with 50g (1¾oz/¼ cup) raisins, spread evenly. Peel, core and slice 1kg (2¼lb) Bramley or other cooking apples; lay the slices over the raisins in the pie dish. Sprinkle the remaining sugar and oat mixture over the apple, and drizzle with the juice of 1 lemon. Put on the top crust and bake in the oven for 30–40 minutes, until golden. Cool on a wire rack before serving.

PEACH PIE Preheat the oven to 180°C (350°F). Line a 28cm (11¼in) pie dish with Vegan Shortcrust Pastry (page 265) and prepare the top crust. Mix 80g (2¾oz/scant ½ cup) soft light brown sugar, 2 tablespoons plain (all-purpose) flour and 1 teaspoon ground cinnamon in a bowl. Put 50ml (1¾fl oz/scant ¼ cup) untoasted sesame oil in a saucepan over a medium heat and add the dry mix, stirring as it thickens. Add the juice of 2 lemons and 1 teaspoon almond extract. Cook for a further 5 minutes, adding more liquid, if needed, to create a sauce. Skin 1kg (2¼lb) fresh peaches by carefully lowering each peach into a pan of boiling water and lifting it out after 1 minute, then lowering it into a bowl of cold water and immediately slipping off the skin. Slice each peach in half, remove the stone (pit), and slice each half into four. Add any escaped juices to the sauce mixture. Arrange the peach slices in the pastry-lined pie dish and pour over the sauce. Add the top crust, pierce it with a fork and bake in the oven for 30–35 minutes. Cool on a wire rack before serving.

RHUBARB TART Preheat the oven to 180°C (350°F). Line a 28cm (11¼in) pie dish with Sweet Press Pastry (page 264) and bake for 15 minutes, as instructed. Put 375g (12oz/3 cups) finely chopped rhubarb in a large bowl, and mix with 50ml (1¾fl oz/scant ¼ cup) oil and the juice of 1 lemon. Mix 80g (2¾oz/scant ½ cup) soft light brown sugar, 50g (1¾oz/⅓ cup) plain (all-purpose) flour, 30g (1oz/⅓ cup) oat flakes (rolled oats and 1 teaspoon ground cinnamon and stir this mixture into the rhubarb for 3–5 minutes. Spread the rhubarb mixture over the pastry case, and bake in the oven for 30 minutes. Cool on a wire rack before serving.

SUMMER FRUIT TART Make the Cool Coconut Crust (page 264) and chill. Wash, trim and halve 250g (9pz) fresh strawberries and 12 seedless grapes. Distribute the fruit halves over the crust. Mix together 25g (1oz) granulated sugar, 1 tablespoon coconut oil and 1 tablespoon lemon juice in a large bowl. Stir briskly for a few minutes to ensure that the sugar is dissolved. Gently stir in 250g (9oz) raspberries, and spoon this mixture over the strawberries and grapes, spreading it evenly in the pie dish. Garnish with a sprinkling of flaked almonds. Chill in the refrigerator for at least 2 hours.

RECIPE FINDER

INDEX

RESOURCES

FAMILY MATTERS

La Leche League International provides info
and data sheets as well as infographics to
support and encourage breastfeeding
https://www.llli.org/breastfeeding-info/

The World Health Organization (WHO)
provides info and data sheets as well as
infographics to support and encourage
breastfeeding
https://www.who.int/docs/default-source/
infographics-pdf/breastfeeding/infographic-
breastfeeding.pdf

THINKING DEEPER

Amateur Beekeepers Association (NSW)
https://www.beekeepers.asn.au

American Beekeeping Federation
https://www.abfnet.org

Australian Honey Bee Industry Council
https://honeybee.org.au

B Corporation: this is an international body
https://bcorporation.net/
https://bcorporation.uk/

British Beekeepers Association
https://www.bbka.org.uk/

British Hedgehog Preservation Society
https://www.britishhedgehogs.org.uk/

Climate emergency information from
the Alliance of World Scientists
https://scientistswarning.forestry.oregonstate.
edu

'Four Changes' by Gary Snyder
https://arthurmag.com/2011/01/31/
four-changes-by-gary-snyder/

Homemade Chocolate Kits
https://www.indigo-herbs.co.uk/shop/buy/
indigo-raw-chocolate-making-kits

https://eu.wholefoodsmarket.com

Private-ownership conservation in Australia
https://www.wildlifelandtrust.org.au/

The Wildlife Trusts
https://www.wildlifetrusts.org/

The Woodland Trust
https://www.woodlandtrust.org.uk/

Support for US forests and woodlands
https://www.forestfoundation.org/about-
american-forest-foundation

Vegan pet foods, advice, product lists,
recipes and suppliers
http://vegepets.info/suppliers.html

GENERAL

Search the Vegan Society Resource pages
https://www.vegansociety.com/

Artisan Vegan Cheeses
https://www.iamnutok.com/our-story

International manufacturer of vegan cheeses
https://violifefoods.com/

ACKNOWLEDGMENTS

I would like to express my gratitude to
Anthony Cheetham and Peter Cox for their
robust commitment to this book; to
Maryanna, for her questions; to Madeleine
O'Shea, for her insightful editing; to Julia
Strauss, for her scholarship.